TRANSFORMING NURSES' ANGER AND PAIN

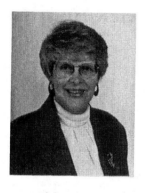

Sandra P. Thomas, PhD, RN, FAAN, is Professor and Director of the PhD Program in Nursing at the University of Tennessee, Knoxville, and teaches in the graduate programs in the College of Nursing. Her initial nursing preparation was at St. Mary's Hospital School of Nursing. She holds bachelor's, master's, and doctoral degrees in education as well as a master's in nursing, with specialization in community mental health. During her doctoral program she majored in educational psychology, with a supporting emphasis in preventive mental health. She has extensive clinical experience, primarily in psychiatric/mental health nursing of adults. She is a member of the American Nurses Association, the American Psychological Association, Sigma Theta Tau International, and the Society of Behavioral Medicine. In 1996 she was named a Fellow of the American Academy of Nursing. She is currently serving a second term on the Board of Directors of the International Council on Women's Health Issues. Dr. Thomas is Editor, *Issues in Mental Health Nursing,* and serves as a reviewer for many other professional journals. Her research has focused on stress, anger, and depression as well as modifiable behavioral variables that affect health. She has presented her research at numerous national and international conferences and has also published extensively. Her previous books are *Women and Anger* (Springer Publishing, 1993) and *Use Your Anger: A Woman's Guide to Empowerment* (Pocket Books, 1996).

Transforming Nurses' Anger and Pain

Steps Toward Healing

Sandra P. Thomas, PhD, RN, FAAN

Foreword by Virginia Trotter Betts

 Springer Publishing Company

Springer Publishing Company, Inc.
536 Broadway
New York, NY 10012-3955

Cover design by Janet Joachim
Acquisitions Editor: Helvi Gold
Production Editor: Kathleen Kelly

01 02/4 3

Library of Congress Cataloging-in-Publication Data

Thomas, Sandra P.
    Transforming nurses' anger and pain : steps toward healing /
Sandra P. Thomas.
        p.   cm.
    Includes bibliographical references and index.
    ISBN 0-8261-1209-9
    1. Nursing—Psychological aspects.   2. Anger in the workplace.
3. Nurses—Mental health.   I. Title.
    [DNLM: 1. Nurses—psychology.   2. Anger.   3. Adaptation.
Psychological.   WY 87 T4615t 1998]
RT86.T48   1998
610.73'01—dc21
DNLM/DLC
for Library of Congress   98-10335
                                                                CIP

Printed in the United States of America

Contents

Foreword

by Virginia Trotter Betts, Past President American Nurses Association

It is both a pleasure and an honor to write this brief commentary on such a timely body of work. Sandra Thomas is and has been a valued colleague of mine for many years as we both work in a variety of leadership roles within the Tennessee Nurses Association. The growing interest by the public and the profession in Sandra's outstanding research on anger has been a joy to watch and has made all of us fellow nurses proud. Now, in this book, Sandra has turned the focus of her work toward us—the nursing profession and the 2.5 million nurses who comprise it.

Nursing is an applied professional discipline that, in addition to knowledge, skill, and critical thinking, requires an intimate relationship with its recipients. Nurses nurse patients at the very times of the patients' lives that are filled with pain, fear, and chaos, and these encounters are frequently laden with stress, sorrow, and intensity. Forget that silly lecture in Nursing101 that said otherwise: The practice of nursing is filled with emotion for both the patient and the nurse. In addition, the world of health care is changing rapidly and its new rules, values, and expectations are confusing everyone. No wonder we come home at the end of even the most productive day with all our nerve endings tingling—we've been nursing!

This book will help nurses better understand one of our very normal feelings—anger—and help us to better evaluate and direct our anger responses. Sandra Thomas's work on anger is now ready to facilitate patient care, not only by nurses better intervening in the anger of patients but also by nurses dealing with their own anger. After reading this book, nurses will be able to see that quality patient care requires an effective contextual presence and that strengthening the community of nursing through self-understanding, professional cohesiveness, and professional collective action is beneficial for every nurse and every nurse's patient.

Preface

I have been to Scutari, to that immense and formidable hospital where Florence Nightingale cared for thousands of British soldiers wounded in the Crimea. As I walked along the dark corridors, the anguished cries of the sick and dying men still rose, reverberating against unfeeling stone. I could see them piled like so many bloody, discarded rags, thrashing and moaning. What consternation Nightingale must have felt upon finding 3,000 men crammed into the Selimiye Army Barracks, which served as the hospital. Four miles of beds, tightly crushed together, held the mutilated bodies awaiting Miss Nightingale's ministrations. The "hospital" had no kitchens, no laboratory, no operating table, no bed linens. It is hard to imagine the conditions at Scutari.

> There were no basins, no towels, no soap, no brooms, no mops, no trays, no plates . . . no knives or forks or spoons. The supply of fuel was constantly deficient. The cooking arrangements were preposterously inadequate, and the laundry was a farce. As for purely medical materials, the tale was no better. Stretchers, splints, bandages—all were lacking; and so were the most ordinary drugs. . . . The very building itself was radically defective. Huge sewers underlay it, and cesspools loaded with filth wafted their poison into the upper rooms . . . the walls were thick with dirt; incredible multitudes of vermin swarmed everywhere. (Strachey, 1996, pp. 16–17)

Have any of us in modern nursing ever faced such appalling conditions? So daunting a task? Compounding the difficulties presented by the sheer volume of work to be done at Scutari was the scathing hostility of the men in authority. The intrusion of Nightingale and her small band of nurses into the all-male military environment was greeted with derision. Obstacle after obstacle was placed before her by the unyielding army bureaucracy. Nightingale also had to deal with conflict and dissension within her own staff. At one point, she began to believe that none of her colleagues had the proper dedication to the work. From this place of filth, horror, and death, a discouraged Nightingale wrote in an early letter home: "There should be a sign: 'Abandon Hope, All Ye Who Enter Here'" (Isler, 1970).

But you know the rest of the story. She did not abandon hope. Enshrined in the lore of nursing history are the incredible achievements of Nightingale at Scutari. Through her energy, vision, and astute management of people and resources, the mortality rate of the soldiers was reduced from 42% to 2% in 6 months. Scutari was transformed into a place of caring, order, and cleanliness. For these remarkable achievements Nightingale was accorded the attributes of near-sainthood. An ideal image of *nurse* entered the psyche of the British people: the gentle "lady with the lamp."

Less well known is the force of Nightingale's anger. Late at night in her little room in the Northwest Tower of Selimiye Barracks, she vented that anger in a torrent of letters that document its extent and force. She minced no words as she described the privations of Scutari to the people back home in England: "No sufficient preparations have been made for proper care of the wounded. Not only are there not sufficient surgeons . . . not only are there no dressers and nurses . . . there is not even linen to make bandages . . . the commonest appliances of a workhouse sick-ward are wanting. . . . (Woodham-Smith, 1951, p. 85). Nightingale passionately advocated for better sanitation, nutrition, and medical care for the British soldiers. Her missives were successful in capturing the attention of the public and kindling their rage as well. For Nightingale, anger was a powerful tool: "I do well to be angry," she said (Strachey, 1996, p. 31).

These words could easily be ours, as we look down the corridors of our own Scutari on the brink of the 21st century. Again, nurses face chaos, vast human need, lack of resources to give proper care, entrenched bureaucracy, and a hostile environment. Today's nurses feel embattled, assaulted, and literally on the firing line. Across the nation, many of us have been victims of the convulsive restructuring of the health care delivery system. As we or our colleagues have been terminated or laid off because of "downsizing" or "rightsizing," unlicensed personnel with minimal preparation have taken our places. Those nurses who remain must do more and more with less and less. Patient safety is a critical issue. Nurses are enraged—justifiably so. Anger spills over to our own peers and takes its toll in fatigue, physical health problems, depression, and substance abuse.

Like Nightingale, can we do well to be angry? Can we transform our anger and pain into something positive? I think we can. Nightingale's words challenge us to "do the thing that is good, whether it is 'suitable for a woman' or not" (Nightingale, 1992). She decried the societal characterization of nurses as self-sacrificing and subservient: "No *man*, not even a doctor, ever gives any other definition of what a nurse should be than this—'devoted and obedient.' This definition would do just as well for a porter. It might even do for a horse" (Woodham-Smith, 1951). Like the founder of modern nursing, today's women—and men—must speak passionately about our concerns. Our anger can be a catalyst for personal and professional empowerment. Let us heed Nightingale's admonition to carry on her fight: "I am now entirely a prisoner in my room from illness; but none the less I cry out to you 'charge, charge! On, on'" (Bishop, 1957).

Introduction

A book is always birthed for a reason. This one is born out of the suffering of many of you, my nurse colleagues, all across America. After hearing your fury and pain in countless workshops and sifting through hundreds of pages of interview transcripts gathered by my research team, I knew that I must write this book. I am convinced that a transformation must take place in nursing, a transformation in the hearts and minds of individual nurses that ultimately creates peace and harmony in our relationships with one another. If we do not link arms to face the challenges presented by a radically revised health care delivery system, nursing's future could be in jeopardy. Nightingale warned us that "no system can endure that does not march." And marchers must be in step with one another.

In this book I share with you what I know about dealing with anger and pain. Some of what I know is from my research, but much of my learning has been acquired in the crucible of tough life experience. I have wrestled with virtually all of the problems in these pages. Bits of my own story are interwoven with fascinating glimpses of the work lives of dozens of other nurses. This book is written to give you hope and confidence that you can surmount the difficulties you are facing. This is a time of fear and uncertainty for nurses. But when bad things happen, better things can be done.

In Part One, we will uncover the causes and consequences of nurses' anger and pain, then move on to more productive anger styles. But emotional healing cannot take place without mending relationships with colleagues, so in Part Two we focus on connecting in deeper, more meaningful ways with other nurses and physicians. Forging alliances with patients is also crucial. Part Three provides a wealth of suggestions to help you transcend the legacy of a painful or abusive past, in order to achieve healing. Caring for the self is a strong emphasis because it is the self that nurses so often sacrifice. Part Four is all about claiming our power, solving the profession's problems, and dreaming our future. I will tell you now that I think our future is a bright one, so this is un-equivocally a hopeful book.

Just a few more words of introduction and then we'll get right to our task. First, let me say that this book is useful for you whether you are male or female. As I wrote it, I was ever mindful that not all nurses are women. Too much of nursing's literature has been addressed to the "sisterhood" of women, ignoring the men in the profession. I have tried to avoid feminine pronouns, but do forgive me if I inadvertently slipped once or twice. Second, let me speak to my use of the term *patients* for the recipients of nursing services. Although debates continue about the proper term (*clients, customers, consumers*), I use the term *patients* for con-sistency. By using this term, I am not implying dependency or lack of ability to enter into a relationship of mutuality with caregivers.

Finally, let me explain my use of quoted material. You will find the words of nurses like yourself leavening the text in every chapter. Unless indicated otherwise, the nurses' words are taken from interview data collected by my research team (see Epilogue for details) or from anger stories shared with me by nurses at workshops or professional meetings. All names appearing in the text are pseudonyms unless individuals gave permission for their real names to appear.

I am grateful to a number of noted nursing leaders from the Ameri-can Academy of Nursing who contributed stories of transforming their own anger and pain. Contributors included Angela Barron McBride, Phyllis Stern, Rosalee Yeaworth, Dixie Koldjeski, Jeanne Quint Beno-liel, Joellen Hawkins, Barbara Barnum, Sharon Valente, Luther Christ-man, and Hildegard Peplau. I thank them for allowing their wisdom to grace these pages.

I

Uncovering Nurses' Anger and Pain

1

Telling Our Stories: What Are Nurses Angry About?

> Anger is a belief that we, or our friends, have been un-
> fairly slighted, which causes in us both painful feelings
> and a desire or impulse for revenge.
>
> *Aristotle, cited in Lazarus* (1991)

American nurses are angry. And they are hurting. Nurses I talk with at conferences and meetings sound more disheartened, cynical, and frightened than ever before. Even during the upheaval created by Medicare's DRGs in the 1980s there was not such widespread distress. I can't remember a time during the past 40 years when there was such pervasive anger among my colleagues. What is fueling all this fury? Listen to the words of nurses:

In ICU your capacity is two patients at the most, because you have fully lined trach-ventilator patients. I walk in, and am told, "We don't have anybody. You're going to have to take these other two patients." And I say to my manager, "This is a very dangerous situation. It's my license you're putting on the line." The only reply I get is, "You do it or you don't have a job."

I've been most angry over the way a patient has been treated. . . . I remember one particular situation and this was a diabetic patient who came for prenatal care. . . to a resident clinic, which is supposed to be overseen by staff physicians. And that just wasn't done in this case. This patient was very brittle and eventually lost the baby. She kept getting different residents

and nobody took that assertiveness to step in and manage her care. . . .
This patient needed that badly. That was the most angry that I believe I've
ever been. I went to the chairman of the department and laid it out. He
said, "Well, we just can't give that kind of one-on-one care to all patients,
you know. This is a patient in the clinic; it's not a paying, private pa-
tient." I was furious.

I had a ridiculous assignment. They were the worst patients on the floor.
Some were on one end of the hall and some on the other end. One was to-
tally confused. One was dying, and I had a lady across the hall who was a
new stroke. Then I had an elderly lady who was 90 years old and who had
just had a fractured hip. I said, "Wait a minute now, I am not an
Olympic sprinter. There's no way I can do all these people." So the secretary
said to me, "What are you doing, causing trouble?"

We had a young patient who died. I was in the room watching the pro-
cedure. No one said anything to the doctor, just "Maybe . . . " or "Have
you thought. . . " or "Could we stop?" I was very angry that day, and I
broke out in a sweat, nauseated. I've never lost control at work like that in
my life, in 14 years, but I did that day. I mean, my heart was racing. The
patient said, "That hurts," and she was told, "No, it doesn't" by the doctor.
That made me angry. I mean, this was just a kid; she was my daughter's
age. I wanted so badly to spit in that doctor's face. I just felt that he had
treated her in such a nonhuman manner. . . . And then, of course, when
she coded, oh, it was like there's nothing that could be done, you know.

The stories of these nurses are just a few of the ones that I, along with
the members of my research team, have collected from nurses across
the country. And there are thousands more who have their own tales of
injustice, outrage, and emotional pain. Undoubtedly, you have some
stories of your own, whether you are a staff nurse, administrator, or educator. I do too. Although it's comforting to know that we're not alone
in our pain, this book is not about bemoaning our lot and licking our
wounds. This book is about doing something positive with our anger.
But first we must explore the nature of the beast. Where it is rational,
we must learn to use it wisely. Where it is irrational or nonproductive,
we must learn to manage it differently. Too many nurses are literally in-
flamed with anger that they cannot manage effectively, and it's burning
them out. The stories I hear disturb and sadden me.

Much of our anger is justifiable. It is kindled in situations that are incongruent with our values and rights as human beings and profession-

als. For example, most nurses value their unique opportunity to be present with the injured, the sick, and the dying, providing empathy and comfort. On the other hand, it is their right to have a reasonable patient assignment so they can give their best to each one. Clearly, the values and rights of nurses were trampled in the examples I selected to begin this chapter. Anger can be a healthy self-protective response in such situations.

However, I am also seeing a lot of nurse anger that is destructive. Whether or not it is justifiable, it's too intense, too prolonged, too punishing—to ourselves as well as to others. In the next chapter, we will look at some of the manifestations and consequences of all this anger. For now, we focus on its causes. Let me warn you that it's grim going in this chapter, because you will be inundated with disturbing material. But bear with me. As in clinical practice, we must assess before we take action.

Why is it important to review the causes, manifestations, and consequences of our anger at this particular time? Haven't nurses always had to deal with the stresses of working in bureaucratic organizations, caring for difficult patients, and spreading themselves thin when they don't have sufficient staff? Indeed, a 12-year-old study ("What *Really* Makes Nurses Angry," 1986) found nurses hot and bothered by things that sound familiar today: short staffing, lack of support from management, paperwork, and poor pay. So what's new in 1998? Emotional distress is *not* new in the nursing profession, but it has *escalated* during the turbulence created by the industrialization of health care in the United States. Although President Clinton's ideas about health care reform were defeated, health care was "reformed" anyway—and not in the way that nurses had envisioned. The name of the game is managed care. It's just about the only game in town now: 74% of American workers are enrolled in managed care plans, as opposed to only 55% in 1992 (Anderson, 1997).

Driven by the exigencies of managed care, the health care system is changing so rapidly that none of us can keep track of all the hospital mergers and acquisitions—$134 billion worth of activity just in the past 4 years (Institute for Health and Socio-Economic Policy, 1996). In fact, every 3 days there is another hospital merger or acquisition (Cahill, 1997). Most often, a for-profit chain like Columbia/HCA buys a nonprofit institution, subsequently eliminating units and services that are not big moneymakers. In some cases, the buyer promptly closes the hospital to reduce competition with others that are in the chain. Such closings can happen with little warning to the employees who are losing their jobs—or to the community that the institution serves. For example, Columbia gave the city of Destin, Florida, just 3 days' notice in 1994 when it closed Destin Hospital (Cahill, 1997).

Whether or not we work in hospitals, all of us in the nursing profession have felt the impact of capitation, competition, and closing of hospital beds and units as the country has been swept by managed care market penetration. We have mastered a whole vocabulary of new words beginning with re-: reengineering, restructuring, redesigning. We have reeled under the unprecedented RN layoffs and job losses in this once-secure profession and watched the deskilling of the workplace in dismay. Not so very long ago, it was common for RNs to make up 90% of the workforce involved in direct care to patients. Today the figure is down to between 65% and 75% ("Staff Nurse Guide to Work Redesign," 1997). To read of the record-breaking profits being made by hospitals (a new high of $13.8 billion in 1994) and the hefty salaries of HMO chiefs (62% higher than salaries of chiefs of other corporations) enrages us, because we who are in the trenches delivering care to patients see firsthand the devastating effects of the corporatization of health services during the past decade (Cahill, 1997; Church, 1997). In a survey by the American Nurses Association involving 1,800 nurses, 80% reported that the quality of patient care declined after RN positions were cut in their facilities (American Nurses Association, 1995). The forecast for the future is cloudy, creating severe apprehension. Fifty-eight percent of registered nurses are the sole support of themselves or their families (Gulack, 1983). What will happen if these nurses lose their jobs?

Nurses are filled with anger as well as fear and consternation about recent events. Let's examine the themes and patterns of nurses' anger that I've observed from Knoxville to Nevada. First, I'll talk about the anger produced by the new trends; then I'll move on to more familiar territory.

"MY WORLD IS TOPSY-TURVY"

Countless studies of human behavior have shown that we are creatures of habit. Change is never easy, especially when the change is unwanted, unanticipated, and profoundly disruptive. Nurses are aghast at the suddenness of the sea change that has engulfed us. Some nurses feel that their whole world is topsy-turvy. A pink slip? It's the last thing they ever would have anticipated. A layoff of their best friend? Unthinkable. When those who survive the personnel cutbacks begin to survey the wreckage of their downsized and restructured institutions, grief is intermingled with impotent rage. "Layoff survivor syndrome" afflicts those who haven't gotten a pink slip yet. I have talked to many nurses who have lost jobs they loved and the comrades-in-arms they had bonded with during many a crisis:

> *I arrived at my unit, ready to go on duty, only to find a posted notice: "Go to 3 West. This unit is closed."*

> *I received a letter [regarding] the change to day shift with a 10-day notice. No managers were available to discuss this. About one and a half hours later I spoke with the medical director, who became offended when I suggested that being spoken to in person would have been a courtesy.*

A recent study (Schilder, 1997) of nurses affected by hospital reengineering found that there were profound personal and professional consequences. Several nurses viewed themselves as "drowning," "treading water," or "hanging by a rope." They saw themselves as victims but were ambivalent about who to blame. They no longer trusted the organization or people who made the decisions. One RN, who had been involved in restructuring committees, viewed the whole process as a farce, because the downsizing decisions had already been made. All of the nurses described the experience as one of the most difficult of their lives. Even those with long employment histories were uncertain about the future, as further reengineering was planned.

As one writer astutely observed, *reengineering* is merely a trendy new term for describing when workers get the shaft (L. Thomas, 1996). Nurses are not the only ones shafted in the reengineering movement. Thousands of American workers have been axed in "downsizing" and "rightsizing" undertaken by corporations to increase their efficiency (and their profits, of course). The reengineering trend was launched in 1993 by Michael Hammer and James Champy with their best-selling book *Reengineering the Corporation: A Manifesto for Business Revolution.* Hospitals, especially those on the East and West Coasts, soon joined the movement, drastically cutting RN positions. Relative to patient volume and acuity level, the number of RNs in American Hospital Association–registered hospitals decreased sharply in 1994 and 1995 (Shindul-Rothschild, Berry, & Long-Middleton, 1996).

When the number of full-time RNs is reduced, the institution usually substitutes temporary nurses or unlicensed assistive personnel (UAPs), a practice known as "deskilling." UAPs are a bargain for a corporation that values profits more than patients: Their pay is less than half that of registered nurses. They can be trained on-the-job in 4 to 6 weeks. But there are no federal or state mandates for content, length, or validation of training of UAPs in acute care settings (Shoffner, 1997). When tasks formerly performed by RNs are assigned to these minimally trained workers, it's pretty scary. Diane Sosne, a Seattle RN, calls it "a dangerous experiment with human subjects" (1996, p. 42). The American Nurses Association and other groups have vigorously protested the increased used of UAPs. As we all know, the patients in today's hospitals are seriously ill or they wouldn't be there. They deserve professional nursing care. Things have gotten so bad that nurses in some institutions would not want their family members to be admitted where they work.

For nursing instructor Amy Crownover, the hospitalization of her father for surgery was a sobering wake-up call. Her diabetic father survived his foot amputation but suffered multiple complications, including bleeding, infection, and problems with his salt and water balance. Amy had this to say about the care he received from UAPs: "Most of the UAPs were kind and caring. They called my dad 'sweetheart,' 'baby,' 'honey.' What they lacked was professionalism and education. They had no assessment skills to catch a small infection before it started draining pus. They took my dad's blood pressure and recorded it faithfully—but had no inkling that the elevated pressure could affect his circulation. In short, the spirit was willing, but the *knowledge* was weak" (Crownover, 1995).

"Weak knowledge" was clearly evident in two appalling incidents reported by a Pennsylvania nurse (Shimer, 1997). Both incidents occurred during hospitalizations of her family member for congestive heart failure and diabetes. In the first, an unlicensed clinical assistant encouraged the patient to drink orange juice and eat crackers after obtaining a blood sugar level of 325. Later, another assistant had the gravely ill woman stand on a scale to be weighed when her systolic blood pressure was only 70. The woman died the next day.

Anecdotal reports of tragedies are reaching the national media, such as the story of hysterectomy patient Rebecca Strunk, who died of peritonitis after her complaints of pain were misinterpreted by UAPs:

Again and again, the 46-year-old mother of two complained of pain in her upper abdomen, and again and again the people who came into her room to care for her wrote down "incisional pain" on her chart. . . . Finally, after three days, as her temperature spiked and her blood pressure plummeted, Strunk's doctors suspected the truth: her bowel had been nicked in the surgery, and she was succumbing to a massive infection spawned by leaking feces. Two days later she died. . . . What made Strunk's case particularly significant was her husband's contention that Strunk died largely because the hospital staff members to whom she described her distress were not registered nurses but "patient-care technicians" who lacked the expertise to interpret her complaints" (Kunen, 1996).

Cutbacks in RN staffing have resulted in forced "floating" and "cross-training" of the nurses who remain on the job. Like medicine, nursing has become highly specialized, and nurses pride themselves on their clinical expertise and technical proficiency within their own specialty area. Nurses are angry about being given responsibilities when they lack the knowledge to assume them. For many years, my specialty area has been psychiatric nursing. I remember my anger when I was pulled from the psychiatric unit one day and assigned a patient who was to have a blood transfusion. Frantically I thumbed through the unit's procedure books to refresh my rusty knowledge (we don't give blood on the psych unit!). This story has a happy ending: I hovered over that patient, paying scrupulous attention to his vital signs, and he had no adverse reaction to the blood. But I remember thinking, "Why am I here? This is crazy! A nurse is not a nurse is not a nurse." So I readily empathized with all of you who told me stories about forced "floating" to units outside your specialty areas. These accounts are illustrative:

I would be floated to orthopedics. . . . given a 5-minute inservice on a complex drain, different kinds of medication, two different pumps—and left with that patient, plus eight other patients. And that really, really, really angered me.

My background was women's health. I'd done intensive care before, but it had been a long time and the particular respirators they were using were different from the respirators I had used.

Cutbacks in RN staffing have also resulted in an increase in the number of nurses suffering injuries on the job. Many of these injuries are caused by lifting and moving patients without adequate help. For example, nurses may see patients attempting to walk and move quickly to assist them. Waiting for additional help to arrive may take too much time. A 12-hospital study conducted by the Minnesota Nurses Association found a 65.2% increase in RN injuries between 1990 and 1992. During that 2-year period, registered nurse positions in the hospitals had been reduced by

9.2%. The majority of injuries were related to either patient transfer (back, neck, and shoulder injuries) or sharps (Helmlinger, 1997).

Then there is the phenomenon of "speedups." While nurses have always been urged to work with speed and efficiency, employer pressures to increase productivity ("speedups" in current lingo) have never been so intense. When told to do more and more with less and less, many of us want to shriek, "Get real! I'm already stretched to the limit!" A majority (65.5%) of the nurses who responded to the 1996 *American Journal of Nursing Patient Care* survey said that the number of patients assigned to them had increased in the past year. Data from this survey, the largest ever conducted on RNs' perceptions of their work life and factors that affect their patients' care, indicated that nurses have less time to comfort and talk to patients, less time to teach patients and their families, and less time to provide basic nursing care (Shindul-Rothschild et al., 1996). One nurse in our own study recounted feeling like a robot "that somebody just pressed the button and said, 'go.' . . . I just felt overwhelmed. I jumped from one room to the next trying to meet these patients' needs. I couldn't do this for this number of patients." Another related,

> *Everybody expected Supernurses. I wanted to live up to the expectation. I tried hard but I would go home frustrated. The patient load was so heavy. I don't feel like I did the care they deserved. I would get really angry.*

Inability to take time for breaks and meals was a common complaint of our study participants. Even skipping breaks, many nurses weren't able to complete their patient care within the specified hours of their shift. Ruefully, they described being called on the carpet for having overtime hours on their time cards. A sense of utter futility at meeting the impossible demands was evident in the words of this nurse we interviewed:

> *I think of the fairy tale Rumpelstiltskin, where they would put the person in the room full of straw every night and say, 'Produce gold!' That's how I feel. I feel like I'm in that room full of straw and I'm being asked to produce gold.*

Bedside nurses are not the only ones experiencing employer demand for speedups, according to the data of the *AJN* survey. Because of cuts in middle and upper management positions, nurse managers are running hard just to stay in place. Almost half of the 7,560 survey respondents reported that their institutions had terminated some nurse managers, and 38% reported the loss of a nurse at the executive level (Shindul-Rothschild et al., 1996).

Nurses in academia are encountering new pressures too. Faculty are expected to pull in research dollars or collect fees for clinical services in addition to their teaching, advising, and publishing. Remember the phrase "publish or perish"? That's not the half of it in today's financially strapped colleges and universities. Many faculty resonate with the it's-so-funny-it-hurts comparison to the pushmi-pullu in a witty article by Judith Vessey and Susan Gennaro (1992). Borrowing from the menagerie of Dr. Doolittle, they selected this two-headed animal to represent the faculty member who must do two sets of tasks at the same time. The greater the amount of pushing and pulling on the beast, the greater the internal dissension and conflict. Vessey and Gennaro predicted in 1992 that the number of pushmi-pullus in the halls of academe would increase exponentially in the tight fiscal environment of modern universities. Already, this prediction has come true, and the pushmi-pullu species is not likely to become extinct in the near future.

Carol Carter has been a nurse educator for the past 5 years, but she still works part time in her clinical specialty area in a hospital. She enjoys caring for the patients but resents the university's failure to give her time to do this work:

They don't give you any time off. Your regular workload is still expected of you. You have to do it on weekends or evening shifts. It makes my evaluation look good, but it makes me angry that we're in a rat race again. Some days it's like I'm between a rock and a hard place. I have all these student papers to grade and school commitments and family commitments. It's running me down. Some days, some weeks I feel angry.

"I AM NOT TREATED WITH RESPECT"

Uncivil or demeaning treatment provokes much anger within the nursing profession. When my research team conducted interviews with nurses, many narratives of being patronized, chastised, and scolded were elicited. Offenders included physicians, supervisors, faculty, and peers. Some nurses attributed such treatment to their age, race, gender, or position in the institutional hierarchy. Others remained bewildered, unable to find any rationale for the disrespectful treatment they received. Mike Evans's story is a good example. Mike is an ICU-CCU nurse with 12 years of experience. He told of a physician who "thrashed me verbally in front of my peers. . . . It was a bizarre reaction on his part. I didn't feel deserving of any criticism. His outburst was totally unprofessional and unwarranted. I really had no idea what had set him off." The incident was especially galling because the "thrashing" took place in front of colleagues.

Bob Hayes's story also took place in the ICU setting, but his attacker was a nursing supervisor, not a physician. Bob's patient had been in an auto accident and had both arms in casts. The physician was examining the casts and the circulation in the patient's fingers, when Bob's supervisor came flying into the unit and started yanking curtains around the patient's bed, berating Bob for violating the patient's right to privacy. Bob relates:

I didn't feel the need [to close the curtains] because the patient was not exposed, there was no procedure. There was nothing going on that would be offensive to anyone. The patient was not bloody or gory. And [the supervisor] comes in and makes this big fuss, embarrasses me in front of the doctor, my coworkers, and the family members. She raised her voice and there was no need for that. She could have called me to the side. Raising her voice made me angry. I was feeling embarrassed and humiliated. I just wanted to clock out and head for the house.

This incident was only one of many that occurred soon after Bob graduated. He grappled with feelings of incompetence when his rigid, stern supervisor continued to criticize his performance, and he thought seriously about leaving the profession: "I almost threw in the towel. I almost quit and went back to K-Mart. But I knew I would be wasting four years of my life." Much has already been written about the crucial transition from the role of nursing student to new graduate. There is plenty of research evidence showing that the graduate experiences "reality shock" (Kramer, 1974), a "crisis of competence" (Cherniss, 1995), and self-doubt. A study of the first year of employment of 180 hospital staff nurses demonstrated that alienation and job dissatisfaction significantly increased by the end of the year (Ahmadi, Speedling, & Kuhn-Weissman, 1987). Support from more experienced nurses could be vital to the novice in that important first year of practice. Yet many new nurses in our study reported they had been treated disrespectfully, adding to their stress. For example, Eve Sanders vividly recalled being "picked on" by an older nurse in her first job as a new graduate: "I was still young, 23. And it was a very intimidating experience. She was a bit older, very pushy, bossy, telling me that is not the right way to make a bed . . . something I had been doing for some time . . . treating me in an infantile manner."

Age is no guarantee of respectful treatment. Joy Carpenter was more than twice as old as Eve when a similar incident occurred during her master's program in midwifery. Despite her maturity and experience, Joy was treated like a child by her preceptor:

> *One time she had assigned me to a patient and told me to manage the labor and everything, and so I did vaginal exams when I thought they were appropriate. She called me aside and reprimanded me and scolded me as if I were a child: "How dare you do that when I am not in the room?" I've done thousands of vaginal exams in my life, and then all of a sudden, because I'm in the student role, I'm not competent to do that anymore.*

Although many of the foregoing stories took place in hospitals, disrespectful treatment of nurses takes place in other locales. Irene Martin is a master's prepared nurse practitioner who performs contract services for a physician. She was appalled when he questioned her invoice for her time:

> *I was very angry because he was not treating me like a professional. He sent me a message through his office manager to tell me that if my invoices were not going to be consistent, then I needed to start to clock in. I can't stand [it when] people question my integrity. I requested to speak to him to discuss the issue, but he didn't want to discuss it with me. When he refused to speak to me, that also made me angry.*

Sexist treatment and sexual harassment were described by both female and male RNs interviewed by our research team. Much more has been written about discriminatory treatment of females, because for most of the profession's history nurses have been female and physicians and hospital administrators male. Florence Nightingale was keenly aware of sexual harassment and noted that "no male hospital administrator or official . . . would intervene on the side of a woman [against] a higher status male, for example a physician or surgeon" (cited in Mrkwicka, 1994). Bullough (1990) called sexual harassment a dominant theme in American nursing, noting how frequently incidents of it were reported in the biographies of nursing administrators and educators. In *American Nursing: A Biographical Dictionary* (Bullough, Church, & Stein, 1988) there are numerous accounts of female nurses running into trouble with male colleagues and either quitting or being fired. When I was in nursing school 40 years ago, I remember how frequently my classmates and I experienced physician harassment, including speculation

about our sex lives and jokes about our bra size. It was not unusual for
doctors to grab our breasts when we were scrubbing for surgery or to
make propositions. Once a psychiatrist exposed himself to me in his office at the mental hospital where we did our psychiatric rotation. Most of
these incidents were shared only with our classmates because no one
dared to confront a powerful male doctor.

When I began to study nurses in 1994, I was hoping to find that
today's nurses were treated with more respect—especially now that sexual harassment is illegal under Title VII of the Civil Rights Act. However,
newer studies document that harassment continues. More than 70% of
female staff nurses surveyed by Libbus and Bowman (1997) reported
sexual harassment. Many episodes involved inappropriate touching, although the chief form of harassment were sexual remarks. Although
nurses become angry at such offensive attitudes and behavior, they still
fear humiliation, retaliation, or job loss if they report the incidents. One
study of nurses found that the greater the nurse's distress, the less likely
she was to report an incident (American Nurses Association, 1993). The
nurse may fear that it is her fault for not setting appropriate limits. She
may not understand what those limits are. Complicating matters is the
unspoken norm on some units that a little flirting is useful in cajoling
irate male physicians. In the ICU, Bob Hayes observed physicians and
nurses "rubbing and massaging each other . . . in an inappropriate, non-
professional way." Similarly, Joy Carpenter related, "I saw other nurses
being touched in ways that were just totally inappropriate . . . physicians
feeling that they had a right to do that . . . Don't ask me how I did it, but
I just knew how to maneuver and get away from them." Greg James re-
sented a female colleague trying to use her "womanly wiles" on him:
"She does it with doctors all the time and they eat it up. I don't. She can't
control me like that. All that did was make me very angry at her for being
so unprofessional. She's a thorn in my side."

Men in nursing certainly have ample justification for anger. Historically, they have experienced rampant discrimination, including insinua-
tions of homosexuality, denial of opportunity to practice in some clinical
settings, and exclusion from the Army Nurse Corps for nearly half a century. They often face the double whammy of being discriminated against
by other men as well as by their female nurse colleagues. Although men
had been prominent in nursing during the Middle Ages and the Renaissance, the modern image of "ideal nurse" was feminized as the Nightingale system of training nurses swept the world. When Christian Hospital
in St. Louis admitted a male nursing student in 1908, the Missouri State
Board declared that the "young man did not fit into the group," and as a

result he left the school (Aldag & Christensen, 1967, p. 375). Despite their chilly welcome, small numbers of men continued to enter the profession, mostly attending all-male schools such as the Mills School of Male Nurses in New York City. Even within schools such as these, men encountered discrimination. Noted nursing leader Luther Christman, speaking of his student days at the School of Nursing for Men of the Pennsylvania Hospital in Philadelphia, remembers:

> *It did not take me long to realize that men were a minority in the profession and were viewed with suspicion by female nurses. . . . I was called a pervert for answering a urologist's request to examine a specimen under a cystoscope while in the presence of a fully draped female patient and female nurse. A similar reaction occurred when I requested a maternity experience. . . . I was denied because of my gender. (Christman, 1988, p. 45)*

Males in nursing are often slotted into specialty areas that are seen as "masculine," such as the emergency department or administration, rather than obstetrics or general floor duty. One man interviewed by Williams (1995) had always aspired to working in OB/GYN but was prevented from participating in that rotation in nursing school and assigned tasks that demanded physical strength instead. Donald Bille went on active duty in the Army Nurse Corps in 1966 after completing his bachelor's degree. He requested the Army's school for public health nursing when he finished basic training. But the first day of the course he was told that the only public health care he could do was changing Foley catheters on the retired Army population, and any care involving women would require a chaperone. He asked for reassignment (Cooper, 1997).

Discriminatory treatment has undoubtedly been a factor in the relatively slow increase in the proportion of men in nursing (currently only about 4% of RNs). Even today, men in nursing hear comments such as, "Surely you're going to pursue your M.D.!" or "Why nursing?" (Brookfield, Douglas, Shapiro, & Cias, 1988). Men who participated in the study by our research team (Brooks, Thomas, & Droppleman, 1996) expressed anger over female nursing colleagues treating them differently because of their gender, calling on them for their "heave-ho-ness" rather than their knowledge. Greg James, manager of a med-surg floor, reported that "if there's anybody heavy to be lifted, even as a manager I would be called to help lift them because I'm a male, instead of the carriers being called." Some men felt excluded from the "sorority" of female nurses and compared themselves to members of other minority groups who are forced to try harder to validate their worth.

Surely African-American nurses will identify with these feelings expressed by the men. Slightly less than 4% of RNs are African-American
(Minnick, Roberts, Young, Marcantonio, & Kleinpell, 1997). Many of
those surveyed in our research endured discriminatory treatment almost on a daily basis. They talked of feeling excluded by the white majority and having to constantly prove themselves. Georgia Preston's
experience was typical:

> *I first started out as an LPN. I was the only African-American woman in
> the class. The instructor tried everything to encourage me to drop out. And
> I recall one OB test that I made 100 on. She just couldn't believe that I
> made 100. She retested me. She said, "I just don't see how you did this." So
> she gave me another test. I made 100 on that one. She never really let up.
> That continued on, through the 13 months. . . . Then a year after that I
> started RN school. . . . I was top in my class. I passed state boards with fly-
> ing colors. And I've been a nurse now for a long time. Everywhere you go
> you have to really prove yourself. If I go to a new hospital, I have to prove
> myself like this is my first day. . . . People judge you just by your color
> alone. . . . When I was with [name of hospital] there were two or three
> black RNs on the floor and we were taking trays in to the patients. Even the
> doctors would say, "Oh there come the girls from the kitchen now." You'd
> have the name tag on, you'd be dressed like all the others; why would you be
> the girl from the kitchen? Sometimes I get so mad I can see fire.*

Elizabeth Barton, who terms herself "young, black, and successful,"
echoed Georgia's complaint of being mistaken for the kitchen help. On
one occasion, although she was the instructor, she was questioned about
being the student. She has also been mistaken for a nursing assistant.
She feels that her colleagues do not respect her. When working with
four white nurses, she was the last to be asked to attempt starting an IV:

> *They'll say something like, "Well, so-and-so tried and she's good." And
> then I'll go in and get it on the first attempt. And that's when they get a
> different opinion of my abilities. It just makes me angry trying to figure out
> why they didn't ask me in the first place. Was it because I was black or was
> it because I was young, or just what factors did they feel made me less ca-
> pable of starting an IV? So most of the time I have to prove myself.*

Fannie Williams, now 58 and a clinical director, recounted a number
of episodes of humiliation and abuse during 31 years of employment at
the same hospital. She sums up the racism she has encountered in her

career: "Racism is like rain; if it's not falling in your location, it's gathering force somewhere nearby."

"I AM BLAMED AND SCAPEGOATED"

As if nurses don't have enough to juggle, just keeping up with their own workload, they also catch the blame for the mistakes and omissions of other health care workers. The lab hasn't drawn the blood, dietary just fed the patient who's NPO, X-ray didn't come to get the fellow whose films were to be done before surgery—and the nurse gets the flak. We've all been there; it's infuriating. Lisa Thompson, a clinical director with 30 years of experience, noted the tendency of physicians to attribute blame to "that stupid bunch of nurses on the floor." She offered the following explanation:

> *I think somebody has to relieve the pressure, has to be blamed, and more often it's nurses. They're quick to be scapegoated. . . . And that's especially true in acute care and labor situations. The physician says he's not responsible—"The nurse didn't call me"—but the nurse reported to him when the first little flicker happened on the fetal monitor. I've seen that quite a bit when physicians were not available. They're quick to let the nurses take the responsibility and take the blame. I think nurses are getting smarter in the way they document and notify, trying to stay out of a bad situation, but there's still a lot of them who do get caught up in a bad situation.*

Joy Carpenter questioned why a doctor couldn't own up to his role in an incident that upset a patient's family: "Why did he have to make *us* scapegoats? I had done everything I was supposed to do and followed the rules. It's like you never know when you're going to get the rug pulled out from under you." Undoubtedly, Mike Evans shared Joy's feeling of having the rug jerked out. He was devastated by a physician's accusation of advancing a Swan-Ganz catheter, which he had not done, although he had no way to prove that he hadn't done it. The situation was especially traumatic for Mike because the physician's accusation replicated a childhood experience:

> *I can still remember a situation when I was barely 6 years old and my [grandmother] found a pair of pants in the living room and went off to my mom raising a big ruckus about how I just stepped out of my pants and left them there. And I hadn't done it. I had no idea how they got there.*

Eve Sanders described being belittled by physicians and yelled at in the hall. When asked what provoked their ire, she related:

Well, I lay it on the line for the patients. I've had physicians be angry with me for telling a patient more than the physician wanted them to know at a particular time. I've borne the brunt of the physician's anger: "Why did you tell her duh duh duh duh duh?" "Because she wanted to know." I have to put myself in the patient's place. I wish I had more guts to confront the physician, to say, "Now look, what you did really hacked me off. You have no right to talk to me that way."

"I FEEL POWERLESS"

Feelings of powerlessness were pervasive throughout the data we obtained from interviews. Nurses wanted someone or something to change, but they did not know how to make that happen. They spoke of their powerlessness in many different situations. RNs were angry about not being involved in the redesign of their units, not having a place at the table when decisions were being made, and not having sufficient resources to do their jobs. Many felt that the work environment could not be controlled. For example, Eve Sanders spoke about her lack of control when ancillary personnel were pulled from her unit by the supervisor: "Basically, my protest was a meek thing, a meek protest. I could not say to the supervisor, 'No, you cannot take my aide.' You know, they did not call to *ask*, they called to *demand*." Carol Carter felt pulled in so many directions that she could not give good patient care:

I knew the stuff I was taught to do, but I did not have time to do it. . . . It is like a rat race. We are here to push pills and drugs, but [we have] no time to do patient care. . . . It seems I always fall behind on time and that makes me angry. . . . It is like you are pulled in 20 different directions. . . . I have no control, no control over the situation.

Lisa Thompson, a clinical director in a large teaching hospital, chafed at closed communication lines and political power struggles:

I have a lot of anger at those higher up in our establishment because I feel as if decisions get made without asking the right people. For Pete's sake, we learn from Japanese [management techniques] that even the person on the line can help with these decisions, but we still are not really doing that. Decisions are made [and] I am perplexed as to how I can make them work.

I'm told, "You have to do it because so-and-so said." Communication lines are often closed that really should be open. And there are still a lot of political power struggles that overshadow what really needs to be done.

Joy Carpenter decried the scarcity of resources: "[Managers] tell you to do the job, but they don't give you the wherewithal to get it done." Bonnie Hartman made a similar complaint: "We don't always have the supplies we need and certainly not the quality because we always get the cheapest—whatever was the lowest bid on the contract." Bonnie, who is in public health, also went on to talk more broadly about "the system" and the capriciousness of decisions that are made on the basis of politics rather than patients' needs:

I get angry at the system—it's that feeling of powerlessness. So many of the things we do in public health are tied to politics. We have money for whatever a particular administration wants us to have. We get a new program because it is a pet project of the governor or, better yet, his wife. We had lots of money for prenatal care during Governor A.'s administration. It was his wife's project. As soon as the administration changed, the prenatal money was gone. Is this really fair to the people we serve?

Often, nurses have the knowledge to remedy a problem but lack the authority to act on it. For example, Ann Smith was well aware that the staffing pattern for her unit was unsafe, but "it took a doctor getting upset to change it and make administration realize that we were functioning unsafely. It's frustrating to me that a doctor has to come and tell [the administration], 'The unit's not safe,' when the nurses are trying to tell that already."

I consider it the epitome of powerlessness when individuals feel that they do not have a voice. A female nursing faculty member lamented:

In my particular work situation we women are absolutely in the minority, a significant minority in a very paternalistic system. It's a "good old boy" system. It's Southern, it's male-dominated, and we are referred to as 'the girls.' We don't get the same ear as a unit that's bringing massive grant money. We just don't have a voice.

"I AM NOT BEING HEARD"

When nurses do try to make their voices heard, too often no one is really listening to them. Geraldine Vincent, an operating room nurse in

Hawaii, has repeatedly requested that her hospital hire aides to help with moving heavy equipment. Although she has been injured on the job twice in the last 7 years, she cannot get her point across: *"There's no acknowledgment that there has been a shift in the type of work we're required to do in the operating room . . . it now requires heavy lifting and moving"* (cited in Helmlinger, 1997).

Not being heard was a common anger-producing experience for the men and women we interviewed. It was a bit of a surprise to the research team that men were just as likely to have this experience as women. Mike Evans spoke of feeling helpless because he was dealing with someone who would not listen. Tom Parker was very frustrated and angry about a chronic problem of heavy assignments. His female colleague always took a lighter load. Over time, this inequity rubbed Tom the wrong way: "Sort of like an ill-fitting pair of shoes. You can get by with them for a while, but soon they're going to rub a sore on your foot, maybe eventually a blister." When he tried to talk with the other nurse, nothing was resolved. She threw up her hands, saying, "I don't need this," and walked off. Her failure to listen *really* made him sore. He said, "I don't like to be just blown off. What I say doesn't necessarily have to be agreed with, but I want it to be considered. I can tolerate inequity to a point if I feel like there's been some kind of communication."

In Linda Harvey's case, it was the charge nurse who failed to listen to her legitimate concerns about a patient's condition. Linda relates:

> *I had a patient who had had a stomach stapling, and something happened that she wasn't absorbing the nutrition. So what the surgeons had to do was go back and redo some of that. . . . After the surgery I was her primary nurse. She got along pretty good, but when she was getting ready to go home, all of a sudden she started having God-awful stomach pain. This woman was not ready to go home. And so I said this to the charge nurse. The charge nurse was a flippant young girl. She said, "There's nothing wrong with her; she's always complaining about stuff." The woman was doubled up with pain, and I was giving her everything I could to try to get her some relief. [The hospital] discharged her, but she was readmitted to another hospital [with] a bowel obstruction.*

Joy Carpenter summed up what it means not to be listened to: "I am most angry at the lack of being heard, that what I need and want does not matter. . . . I am a nonentity. . . . I would like the courtesy of being heard."

"I AM NOT GETTING ANY SUPPORT"

Lack of support was one of the most poignant aspects of nurses' anger stories. Joy Carpenter remembered the sarcastic retort of her night supervisor when she called to ask for help: "I needed help desperately in labor and delivery. The night supervisor said, 'Well, where do you think I'm going to get these nurses, cut out paper dolls?' " Linda, speaking of nurse administrators, asserted that "I have never seen where they will be your advocate. They sell you down the tubes. They have totally lost sight of the nursing side. And you shouldn't be at sides or at war." Many nurses spoke in the language of war as they talked about their work. They used an incredible number of military metaphors and similes: "It's like being on the firing line"; "We feel sabotaged"; "It's like an armed camp"; "We really don't know how to fight back"; "I don't know if I'll ever muster all that it takes." It became clear to the research team that nurses yearned for some allies in their daily battles. They especially wanted affirmation from managers. But affirmation is not what they got.

Nurses were angry because they were always being told what they were doing wrong. No one mentioned what they were doing right. A woman in one of my anger workshops described her first evaluation conference on a new job. Her supervisor told her only negative things. "Much to my embarrassment, I cried," she told me. "I felt bad with no positive affirmations." Bob Hayes provided a graphic description of his autocratic nurse manager who walked through the unit "like a stick stirring up rattlesnakes," getting all of the nurses "in an uproar and tense . . . pointing out these small things. . . . She would only let you know when something was wrong. And that was quite frequently, in her opinion." Sue Green believes she is doing some good things, but "nobody will remember it."

The longing for support was evident in stories of nurses at all educational levels (from AD to PhD) and at many diverse practice sites (from inpatient oncology to outpatient primary care clinic). Eve Sanders was the first nurse practitioner in an obstetric practice. She displayed considerable fortitude in remaining on the job in the initial months when she received absolutely no support from the older physicians in the group: "They literally did not talk to me for a year—except to find fault: 'You didn't tell [the patient] this or didn't tell her that, or you didn't reassure her well enough.' "

Although a few nurses described a coworker who could be counted on for an encouraging word or a hug, most did not seem to have a workplace support person. Competition and mistrust were more frequently described. Sue Green ruefully acknowledged, "One of the biggest voids in my life is peer support." Many nurses were reluctant to ask for support from others, even from those they trusted. It was not unusual for a nurse to be going through a life-changing event of major proportions, such as a divorce, without sharing the news. This reluctance to ask for collegial support is common in the helping professions, because the usual (and more comfortable) role is giver of help, not receiver of it. Asking for support is somehow equated with inadequacy or weakness. Nurses say they do not want to burden others. Carol Carter explained: "I was brought up that you don't burden other people with your problems. I'll be there for someone else, but it's like I don't feel as if I have the right to burden other people with my problems."

I contend that it's time to lay down some of our burdens. Most of us, as revealed in the stories throughout this chapter, are carrying a heavy load of anger. The rest of this book is devoted to the unpacking and transformation of that anger. Some of the work we must do alone, because only we know exactly how we got all that stuff packed in the bag. But we cannot do all of the work alone. We need to enlist some helpers. In some cases, they may be friends, family, or therapists, but remember that your nurse colleagues will have the best grasp of the unique anger provocations in this profession of ours. Don't leave them out. As you do the assignments listed under "Steps Toward Healing" in every chapter, find a partner or a support group to go on the healing journey with you. The bag won't be nearly as heavy if its load is divvied up. In my view, we cannot give the care that society needs us to give to hurting people unless we care for *ourselves,* which includes acknowledging and acting on our real feelings, and care for *each other,* which includes making a daily effort to be supportive to our colleagues.

As Lynda Carpenito expressed it: "When you go out in the nursing world, hold hands before crossing the street and stick together."

2

Exposing the Consequences of Mismanaged Anger

Nurses don't feel good about the ways they handle their anger, and I'm concerned too. While anger in itself is neither good nor bad—and it *can* be used to accomplish good things—much of it is hidden or mismanaged. Although some nurses told our research team that they screamed or discharged anger in motor activity (by throwing charts, hitting doors with fists, or stalking off from an offender), they seldom felt relief from such actions. Instead, they were ashamed of losing control. More commonly, angry feelings were stifled or somatized, held inside the body until the nurse had a splitting headache or upset stomach. The consequences of mismanaged anger include fatigue, depression, addictions, even hypertension and cardiovascular disease, and I will cite plenty of research evidence shortly. What I am saying is that anger can make you sick. Think of the last time you "swallowed" your anger at work and it sat there all day like a greasy doughnut, heavy in your stomach. The anger may have caused you to have heartburn: Anger does "hurt around the heart," as one of our research subjects told us (Thomas, Smucker, & Droppleman, in press). And if anger becomes chronic, it may be propelling you along the path to burnout, that unhappy state in which you feel like saying: "Take this job and shove it!" Some of the responses to the AJN Patient Care Survey (Shindul-Rothschild et al., 1996, pp. 30–31) suggest that this is a national epidemic:

> I work at a "prestigious" medical center. I am unable to give good care to my patients. The turnover rate increases but nothing is done. It's making me want to leave nursing!

Nursing, as I first worked in it, no longer exists. It's become a business, with profit the bottom line and patient care a very low priority. I will leave nursing soon and never look back.

Nursing morale is at an all-time low. I plan to leave nursing in the near future, and I can't wait! . . . I shudder to think of what the future of nursing holds.

THE ANGER-BURNOUT LINK

What is burnout? How did these nurses get that way? Could this happen to you? Burnout is a familiar term, but most of us have not stopped to consider its complexity. It is a phenomenon that involves stress, although it is not synonymous with stress. Undeniably, nursing has always been a stressful occupation, but not all of us burn out. Research shows that the type of nursing unit doesn't matter either. Whether we work in intensive care, medicine, surgery, or psychiatry units, some of us burn out, but others do not (Duquette, Kerouac, Sandhu, & Beaudet, 1994). Nor is the burnout syndrome equivalent to depression; it is more like emotional exhaustion (Jones, 1982). Maslach (1982) described three phases of burnout. In the first, individuals begin to experience the emotional exhaustion. They feel drained. Next, they develop negative ideas about their patients, coworkers, and themselves. Finally, there is the phase of total disgust. While burnout is not considered an illness, a burned-out nurse could become physically or mentally ill if the condition persists over time (Duquette et al., 1994).

What starts the process of burning out? I have a colleague who observed that burnout is *not* likely to occur in those nurses who have never been "on fire," and I think the literature proves her right. The syndrome tends to afflict highly idealistic professionals who begin their careers "on fire" with the desire to provide compassionate help to others. These individuals become overly involved in their work and overly burdened by the needs of their patients. Eventually, they begin to doubt their competence because they can't keep up with the demands. The metaphor of being engulfed by fire is alluded to by one nurse who is burning out: *"I hate coming to work because I feel [that] once I'm here it engulfs me like fire"* (Larson, 1987). It makes sense that nurses who feel this way may begin to distance themselves emotionally from patients as a survival tactic. Unfortunately, they feel even worse for doing so, blaming themselves for not being able to enact their idealized image of the "good nurse" (Larson, 1987).

Cary Cherniss (1995) conducted a valuable study of teachers, lawyers, therapists, and public health nurses, documenting their loss of idealism in the first year of practice. All had approached their work with unrealistic expectations of themselves and their clients. When confronted with uninterested students and noncompliant clients, many began to doubt their own competence and blame themselves for failing to accomplish what they had set out to do. For example, public health nurse Sarah Prentiss was distressed when an older woman told her, "I don't know why you're bothering with me. I just want to die" (Cherniss, 1995, p. 19). Sarah took this client's statement personally, asking herself, "Gee, what's wrong with me? . . . I might have done something wrong. Maybe I just turned her off. Maybe it was just a personality conflict. But I didn't see it, and that's the thing that bothered me—that I didn't have enough insight to see the problem" (Cherniss, 1995, pp. 19–20). Sarah did not consider that her client was weary of illness and poverty, nor did she acknowledge that even the most seasoned, highly skilled professionals are unable to motivate some clients to change their attitudes and behaviors. She eventually left public health nursing.

Sarah is one of those nurses who will be found in turnover statistics. Leaving is the most commonly selected solution: leaving the problems, leaving the agency, or leaving the profession. But some who burn out do not leave. You can find them in every workplace, disillusioned and disengaged but sticking around because they see no alternative. Some don't know where else to go—or whether they can handle the stress of job hunting or going back to school. The barriers to leaving are undeniable for many: They and their families cannot do without the income, and even a temporary disruption in salary would be disastrous to their financial status. For public health nurse Jessica Andrews, staying in her job was mainly a matter of economics:

> *Unfortunately, my divorce was final in June. That's another reason I'm staying at the health department and doing what I'm doing. . . . I need the insurance, I need the pay. . . . I don't want to go through the risks of setting up my own business right now. I want Blue Cross, and I want orthodontic care and eyeglass care and all that. And you can't do that privately." (Cherniss, 1995, p. 60)*

Where does anger fit in the burnout picture? Difficulty handling anger can be a critical predisposing or precipitating factor in burnout. In a recent study of 297 hospital nurses, researchers found that those with high burnout scores reported the greatest amount of conflict with other nurses and supervisors (Hillhouse & Adler, 1997). Another study showed that anger directed at the self was more strongly correlated with burnout than anger directed toward others (Firth, McKeown, McIntee, & Britton, 1987). These correlational studies do not make it clear whether anger leads to burnout or is a byproduct of it. But using logic, an argument can be made that frequent job-related anger predisposes an individual to burnout. Take the case of the perfectionist. Fran Erwin, one of our study participants, is a good example. Fran told us, "Performance equals approval; performance equals worth." It makes sense that if a nurse approaches his or her work with a high degree of perfectionism, a lot of anger is going to be generated—at others for making errors and at oneself for failing to achieve perfection. If the anger often erupts in conflictual interactions with others, it can drive away that nurse's potential sources of support. Even if it is not verbally expressed, sitting on a lot of anger certainly has the potential to sour one's own attitude toward the job.

Thinking of perfectionism and its link to anger brings to mind our study (Thomas & Jozwiak, 1990) of female nurses who were either Type A (a hard-driving behavior pattern linked to coronary heart disease and other morbidity) or Type B (a more easy going behavior pattern). Researchers have found the Type A pattern prevalent in nurses: In one study, 82% of a sample of staff and head nurses classified themselves as Type A (Cronin-Stubbs & Velsor-Friedrich, 1981). As researcher Sharol Jacobson noted, "We do not know whether Type A persons become nurses or whether nursing turns people into Type A personalities, but both literature and observations of nurses from many settings support the prevalence of the pattern among nurses" (Jacobson, 1983, p. 38). At any rate, my colleague John Jozwiak and I were interested in exploring the differences between Type A and Type B nurses. We asked the nurses to fill out a Type A questionnaire and to describe themselves in response to the question "Who am I?" on an unstructured paper-and-pencil test called the Twenty Statements Test (TST).

Here's what we found: Type A nurses scored significantly higher than Type Bs on the questionnaire items about intense job involvement, speed/impatience, and competitiveness. They also described themselves quite differently than Type Bs in response to the question "Who am I?" on the TST. John and I sorted the 1,202 TST responses of Type A and Type B nurses and coded them into categories. The Type A nurses were more likely to describe themselves as compulsive and perfectionistic. They viewed time as an enemy (e.g., "I often do too many things", "I cannot find time to play tennis", "I'm busy all the time", "I would like to manage time better"), in contrast to their Type B counterparts, who did not feel such extreme pressure.

To John and me, the most striking difference between Type A and Type B nurses was in the prevalence of self-aggrandizing responses on the TST. Self-aggrandizement characterized 73% of Type A nurses, compared with only 23% of Type B nurses. Type A nurses used descriptors such as "charming," "go-getter," "talented," "important," "beautiful," and made frequent references to their leadership roles or position titles, while Type Bs said, "I'm a good nurse" or "I'm a good worker." Type As evaluated themselves more favorably than others ("I see the need for self-improvement in those around me", "I am the stronger force in my marital relationship"), whereas this tendency was not evident in Type B responses (Thomas & Jozwiak, 1990). In summary, the Type A nurses appeared to be engaged in competition with time and themselves, as well as in competition with other people.

While this study did not examine anger variables, it is easy to see that Type A nurses are bringing some attitudes and behaviors with them to the workplace that could kindle angry emotion. The competitiveness and self-aggrandizement of Type A nurses could contribute to problems in interpersonal relationships with coworkers. It stands to reason that people with a high need to prove that they are important or superior to others may be threatened by anyone claiming to be comparably important. To the extent that Type As feel compelled to point out their coworkers' faults and needs for self-improvement, there is a strong likelihood of hostile exchanges and resentment. After all, who likes to receive pointers about their faults?

There are other adverse consequences of Type A. The sense of urgency could lead the Type A nurse to view less driven individuals as lazy or unproductive—and to view much-needed rest and recreation as "wasting time." Furthermore, Type A nurses are setting themselves up for considerable frustration and anger if they expect speed and efficiency in bureaucratic work environments. As we all know, bureaucratic functioning can be tediously slow.

Self-Assessment

Are you on the path to burnout? Take a few minutes and respond to these questions:

1. Do you feel discouraged about work and often think about quitting?
2. Do you feel irritable and angry on the job?

3. Have you noticed more difficulty getting along with your co-workers?
4. Have you lost interest in the patients? (If you teach, substitute *students.*)
5. Have you felt fatigued during the workday?
6. Have you missed work lately due to colds, flu, or other minor illnesses?

If you answered yes to several of these questions, you probably need to rekindle your flame. Read on for some burnout remedies.

Steps Toward Healing

1. Relinquish perfectionism. In the study by Cherniss (1995), the professionals who were least likely to recover from burnout were those who set unrealistic goals for themselves. Adjust your expectations for yourself—and for those you work with. We all have limitations and vulnerabilities. We all make errors; they are excellent learning experiences.
2. Acquire conflict management skills. Nurses need to know how to negotiate and "work the system." However, few of us learn how to do this in nursing school. Negotiating skills can be learned in continuing education courses and practiced in workshops. Instead of leaving your unit for greener pastures, try to bargain for needed changes. Recruit some colleagues to join you, make a plan, then act.
3. Ask for a change in assignments. If you no longer feel that your work is enjoyable—and there is no hope of negotiating to bring about a more satisfactory state of affairs—consider a change. Research shows that a change in job assignments every 5 years or so is a good way to keep up people's enthusiasm for their work (Pelz & Andrews, 1966).
4. Focus on the intrinsic rewards of nursing. In the movie *Jerry Maguire*, the protagonist urges his client, a football player, to reflect on what football was like for him when he first started playing, to remember what he loved about the game before he became focused on the money and the trappings of success. Likewise, I ask you to think back to your motivation for entering nursing. What was it that led you to pursue such a difficult course of study? What was it that you really loved to do? Try to recapture that initial excitement. Marks (1979) pointed out:

Our energy tends to become fully available for anything to which we are highly committed, and we often feel more energetic for having done it. We tend to find little energy for anything to which we are not highly committed, and doing these things leaves us feeling "spent," drained, and exhausted. (p. 31)

THE ANGER-DEPRESSION LINK

Burned out, angry nurses are not so hard to identify. Most know how they feel and readily verbalize their disillusionment with their work. But depressed nurses are not always aware that they have become depressed. Alfred Adler (1956) called depression the "silent temper tantrum." Its onset is insidious—it can sneak up on you. That is exactly what happened to a friend of mine last summer. She didn't know she had suffered from depression. She had no idea what was wrong. Although she had always loved people, it seemed to require too much effort to get out and see them. She was intelligent and well educated, but concentration was difficult, and she kept forgetting things. She didn't have the energy for her usual physical activities: Her swimsuit hadn't been wet in months, and her NordicTrac had gathered dust. One day I told her I thought she was depressed. After a thorough examination, her doctor came to the same conclusion and prescribed antidepressant medication. She's much better now.

My friend's experience is typical of many women. She learned early in life that her own needs were not important, that she was destined to give care to others. Her first thought in any situation is tending to the needs of those around her. When others are not happy, she assumes excessive responsibility for their unhappiness and intensifies her efforts to make things right. She takes on others' stress and worries, doing their worrying for them. Even when she is tired and would like to rest, she finds it very difficult to say no. She would feel guilty if her "no" caused disappointment. And she takes the blame for the failure of her marriage, although her former husband was a self-centered man whose unhappiness could not have been assuaged, no matter what she did to love and please him. After their divorce, she was down on herself rather than angry at him.

Not surprisingly, my friend selected a profession in which she nurtures, with a maternal-child specialty. She has always "given at the office" and given at home too. Not surprisingly, her role socialization as a woman and as a nurse to be a selfless, ever-nurturing, mother figure placed her at risk for greater stress and depression. Some researchers speak of depressive symptoms as the "cost of caring" for women (Turner & Avison, 1989).

Statistics consistently show that women's risk for depression exceeds that of men by 2 to 1. Although female gender role socialization plays a part in increasing that risk, no single theory or set of predisposing factors provides a complete explanation of the 2:1 ratio. Depression involves biochemical change, but no one knows if the chemical changes in the brain *cause* depression or *result* from depression. We do know from research that demographic characteristics make little difference in the likelihood of becoming depressed. Depression afflicts women of all income and educational levels and claims as its victims white, black, Asian, and Hispanic women. Depression can occur whether a woman is married or unmarried, employed or unemployed (McGrath, Keita, Strickland, & Russo, 1990).

Looking at the interaction of a woman's work and family roles has proved to be useful in recent studies on risk for depression. If married women worked but had low marital strain and low job strain, they had the lowest rates of depression. Unmarried working women with low job strain also had low rates of depression. Who had high rates? Employed wives with high marital strain *and* high job strain. However, being employed was better than being unemployed for women with high marital strain; at highest risk for depression was the unemployed wife with high marital strain (Aneshensel, 1986). Motherhood further complicates the picture, especially for working moms who have sole responsibility for child care and difficulties arranging for it. These women have extremely high depression levels (Ross & Mirowsky, 1988). The age and number of children make a difference too. As you might suspect, the risk of depression is higher for mothers of young children, and the risk increases with the number of children living at home (Radloff, 1975). Mothers with children younger than 5 years old who don't have a supportive partner are more apt to become clinically depressed than any other group of adults (Carroll, 1993).

The connection between anger and depression has been probed by researchers. Commonly, it is believed that holding anger in leads to depression. You probably remember the depression-is-anger-turned-inward hypothesis from nursing school. There is support for this hypothesis in a number of older studies (Biaggio & Godwin, 1987; Friedman, 1970; Lemaire & Clopton, 1981), as well as in a newer study conducted by Joyce Bromberger and Karen Matthews (1996). They followed 460 middle-aged women for 3 years and found that introspective, passive women who held their anger in were indeed more prone to bouts of depression. Why is this so? Here is my explanation: When anger is not expressed, injustice cannot be remedied and interpersonal conflicts cannot be resolved. Then women ruminate about the issues that made them angry in the first place, prolonging and increasing the bad feelings. Women are more likely than men to ruminate after negative events, whereas men tend to distract themselves by doing something physical, such as playing a sport (Nolen-Hoeksema, 1987).

The anger-turned-inward view of depression has been challenged. There is a body of literature showing that overt, confrontive expression of anger is also associated with depression (Billings & Moos, 1985; Folkman & Lazarus, 1980; Weissman & Paykel, 1974). Carol Tavris, who sparked much debate with her book *Anger: The Misunderstood Emotion*, contended that "[:] If anything, anger is depression turned outward. Follow the trail of anger inward, and there you find the small, still voice of pain" (1989, p. 14). A woman who participated in one of our own studies told us: *"Through counseling I've learned that I handle depression by being angry. . . . I would lash out at everything and really didn't know why. . . . I had all this anger to work through and to understand."*

What can be concluded from all of this? Whether depression is anger turned inward or anger is depression turned outward, the bottom line is that anger clearly plays a significant role in depression. In the Women's Anger Study, our own research team found that depressed women definitely have greater levels of anger than women who are not depressed. They manage this anger in both of the unhealthy ways we have talked about so far: turning it inward and venting it outward in harsh attacks on others (Droppleman & Wilt, 1993). Our studies of anger in nurses, whether female or male, suggest that nurses are at risk for depression because they have high levels of anger and use the same unhealthy anger management styles. A study by my colleague Kathryn Skinner found a sizable 27% incidence of depression among female registered nurses working at a metropolitan hospital (cited in Little, 1991). This figure is higher than the 20% to 25% incidence of depression in community samples (McGrath et al., 1990).

What about depression in male nurses? I located only one study that compared levels of depressive symptomatology in female and male nurses. Its conclusion was unexpected: The male nurses had higher levels than females (Firth et al., 1987). Some 37% of the men were mildly or moderately depressed, as compared to 28% of the women. The incidence of depression in the male nurses was significantly higher than the incidence in males in the general population, which was only 10%. This British study needs to be replicated in the United States.

Self-Assessment

Despite the knowledge you acquired about depression in nursing school, you may not be aware that you, or perhaps your colleagues, have symptoms and need treatment. Depression can occur in mild, moderate, or severe forms. While severe symptoms such as psychomotor retardation are likely to be noticed by family members and coworkers, more subtle manifestations such as appetite change may escape their notice. You yourself may not attribute your weariness and loss of interest in things to depressive illness. Have you experienced five or more of the following symptoms during the past 2 weeks?

Depressed mood most of the day
Diminished interest or pleasure in activities
Weight loss or weight gain
Insomnia or hypersomnia
Psychomotor agitation or retardation
Fatigue or loss of energy
Feelings of worthlessness or guilt
Diminished ability to think or concentrate
Thoughts of death or suicide

If you have five or more of these symptoms (at least one of which is either depressed mood or loss of pleasure) and you do not have hypothyroidism or other medical conditions, you may be experiencing a major depression (American Psychiatric Association, 1994). Other symptoms will be evident in a person with bipolar disorder (manic depression) or psychotic depression; these conditions will not be dealt with here.

There is another disorder that we need to mention. Some individuals suffer from a more chronic kind of depression: dysthymic disorder. The symptoms are similar to those listed above for major depression but are less severe. In fact, the symptoms are so much a part of the person's day-to-day experience that they usually go unreported to health care providers. People with dysthymic disorder often say, "This is just how I am," meaning that it is "normal" for them to be self-critical and unhappy. The most common symptoms of dysthymic disorder are feelings of inadequacy, generalized loss of interest or pleasure, social withdrawal, feelings of guilt about the past, irritability or anger, and decreased activity or productivity. Have you experienced depressed mood for most of the day, for more days than not, for at least 2 years? Along with the depressed mood, have you noted symptoms such as these? If so, then you may have dysthymic disorder (American Psychiatric Association, 1994).

While mental health professionals continue to debate the cutoff separating subclinical and clinical levels of depression, I believe that even subclinical depression deserves prompt attention. Moderately depressed persons may have significant problems keeping up at work (Nolen-Hoeksema, 1990), and if they manage to get through the workday, they fall into bed, exhausted, when they get home. I have, in fact, known a number of nurses who worked their shift, ate, slept, and returned to work, engaging in no recreation or social interaction. The quality of their lives was greatly diminished. They were depressed but did not realize it.

If you are depressed, you need to see your health care provider. A visit is urgent if you are preoccupied with thoughts of death or suicide. Be aware that both medication and psychotherapy have proven to be effective. However, I recommend psychotherapy along with antidepressants because there is a high risk of relapse (as much as 60%) with medication alone (Antonuccio, Danton, & DeNelsky, 1995). You will feel better about yourself when you are learning principles that will help insulate you from later episodes of depression (Yapko, 1997). The good news about depression is that it can serve an important adaptive purpose, permitting resolution of a deadlock in functioning and leading to learning and growth (Gut, 1989). Out of depression, you can emerge more psychologically whole. There are a number of self-management techniques that you can begin to use. In addition to managing your anger more effectively, which is addressed in a later chapter, try the approaches listed below.

Steps Toward Healing

1. Stop blaming and criticizing yourself when you have not met every patient's or student's needs. Instead, focus on the people you have helped and the things you have done well each day. Beck (1976) has pointed out that the failures of those who are depressed are no more severe than the failures of nondepressed individuals: It is how they interpret their failures that differs. As you review your day, make sure you affirm yourself for at least *one good thing*. I try to do this while driving home from work. For example, I might say to myself, "If I hadn't been there today, that student wouldn't have had a shoulder to cry on." When Ann Peden (1996) studied recovery from depression, her study participants emphasized the importance of positive affirmations:

I try to put a positive thought in when I start having negative ones, and I use writing affirmations and keep a lot of scrap paper. . . . I just write over and over again.

I had some positive affirmations that I had memorized. I've got them written on index cards. I had them pasted up around the house.(p. 293)

2. Learn to tolerate ambiguity. Psychologist Michael Yapko (1997) claims that this is the most important skill to ward off depression. According to Yapko, it is in response to ambiguity that many individuals make negative interpretations that can lead to depression. In most life situations, there is no single correct answer but a variety of possibilities. As Yapko puts it, "Life is inherently ambiguous; an experiential Rorschach" (p. 75).
3. Find an activity to distract yourself from rumination. Physical activities work best because they lead to the release of endorphins that lift your mood. Walk, swim, or garden. Make yourself get off the couch and go outside. And make yourself call a friend to join you. You need to be with people. I know it's hard, but you'll be glad you made the effort.
4. If you have experienced a loss of a valued relationship through death or divorce, you do need to mourn the loss. Your depression is the result of mourning that was never completed. Give yourself permission to cry or be angry. Let the guilt go. There is a wonderful book that I have recommended to countless friends and clients: *How to Survive the Loss of a Love* by Colgrove, Bloomfield, & McWilliams (1991). Buy yourself a copy. You *can* survive this loss and you *can* have other relationships.
5. Even while depressed, there are always some times of day when you feel better. Use those times to engage in activities that you used to enjoy before you became depressed. How long has it been since you treated yourself to a luxurious bubble bath or bought yourself a totally frivolous gift? Build more pleasure into your life. This is a time to care for yourself with the same loving devotion you give to so many others.

ANGER'S LINK TO PHYSICAL SYMPTOMS

Let's turn our attention to the physical effects of angry emotion. As a nurse, you already know that anger produces a powerful physiological arousal. To briefly review, the cerebral cortex signals both the adrenal medulla, which secretes adrenaline and noradrenaline, and the adrenal cortex, which secretes cortisol. The heart pounds harder and faster, blood pressure rises, respiration increases, and fat cells release fat into the bloodstream (which is converted to cholesterol unless burned up in intense exercise). The arteries carrying blood to the skin, kidneys, and intestines constrict, and the arteries to the muscles dilate. The body is primed to take action. Stevick (1971) described it as a "wanting-to-burst-forth body" (p. 144). When this strong arousal is not dissipated in action of some kind, a variety of bodily discomforts can result: tense muscles, headaches, GI upsets, and just plain fatigue—that bone-tired, wiped-out feeling when you are not sure you can put one foot in front of the other to walk out to the parking lot at the end of a day's work.

Research in the new field of psychoneuroimmunology (PNI) shows that anger even affects the functioning of the immune system. PNI scientists have identified 60 to 100 biochemical messengers (neurotransmitters, neuropeptides, growth factors, and lymphokines) that link emotional states with the immune system. Therefore, emotions are not contained in the mind or brain, but are "out there" throughout the body as well. The autonomic nervous system directly relates to lymphocytes and macrophages. One study documented significant inhibition of salivary IgA—the first line of defense against pathogens in the upper respiratory tract, the GI system, and the urinary tract—for 5 hours after experiencing anger (Rein, Atkinson, & McCraty, 1995). Not surprisingly, another study found that the common cold was linked to increased anger and tension during a 4-day period prior to the onset of symptoms (Evans & Edgerton, 1991). It appears that the subjects' emotional state lowered their resistance to the cold virus. I know that many of you can attest to anger's deleterious effects from your own experience. Consider the words of a Florida nurse quoted in the February 1995 issue of American Journal of Nursing (1995):

> *We have colds, flu, people are just worn down. You constantly see runny noses on the units. Lots of tension, tension headaches. We eat Tylenols. . . . All of this under the guise of health care reform. They spend $7 million in computer software . . . but they can't hire nurses."*

Not only tension headaches but also migraines are connected with anger. Georgia Witkin, a psychiatry professor in New York, has presented case material of a patient who feared her own angry impulses and suppressed them: "Rosemary knew that her migraine attacks always followed situations in which she was enraged but felt that she couldn't express her anger. She claimed that she had had years of 'nonassertive-ness training,' and feared that showing her anger would destroy her image as the patient wife and mother" (Witkin, 1991, p. 57). Research supports Dr. Witkin's clinical material. In an interesting study comparing the reactions of female migraine patients and women without migraines in an anger-provoking situation, researchers found that the migraine patients tended to suppress their anger. Expressive behaviors, such as pounding the table, occurred more often in the women without migraines (Grothgar & Scholz, 1987).

Some of the participants in the Women's Anger Study understood the connection between suppressed anger and physical symptoms. In fact, the particular symptom often aptly expressed their feelings. A nurse who told us she "had the experience as a nurse of being voiceless, of having no voice" realized that she often developed a sore throat when she became very angry about work-related matters over which she felt she had no control. Another woman (not a nurse) displayed remarkable insight in the following narrative:

> *I very much believe in the mind/body connection. . . . I can think of specific examples . . . when something was happening that I just couldn't stand and then that's the way I'd express it—I had lower back pain and I couldn't stand up straight. Then there was another time when I wanted to tell someone something that bothered me and I just couldn't bring myself to do it. I got laryngitis and couldn't talk. . . . Then . . . there was some project [my husband] wanted to just bulldoze through. I like to do projects, but I'm kind of meticulous. I take my time and do it slowly. . . . He was pushing us through . . . and my neck started hurting. It's a "pain in the neck," you know.*

Self-Assessment

Tuning in to your own bodily sensations of anger is important. In times of stress and anger, most of us have a particular organ or system that seems to get the brunt of it. Take a few minutes to think about your most common somatic symptoms. Do you get a severe headache? Do you get a knotted feeling in the stomach? Do you become constipated? Do your neck and shoulders tighten? Noted holistic nurse Leslie Kolk-meier (1995) recommends a simple technique called body scanning that you can use to assess muscle tension:

> *It has been estimated that we spend 40 minutes a day, or at least 2 years of our lives, waiting. We can choose to spend this time simply waiting (and*

probably growing impatient, thus adding to our tension burden), or we can use it to scan our bodies for muscle tension. Body scanning is taking a moment to inventory all parts of the body mentally and identify areas that are full of tension. (p. 584)

Once the tense areas are identified, a relaxation procedure can be used. You can do this during the workday when the person at the other end of the telephone line has placed you on hold, when you are waiting for an elevator, and anytime you have a free minute or two. When this practice becomes part of your daily routine, the buildup of extreme tension can be avoided.

Steps Toward Healing

1. Value the feedback your body is giving you. The wisdom of the body was greatly respected by our ancestors, who listened more closely to its cues. We tend to consider bodily aches and pains as mere annoyances that must be banished with chemicals—instantly, if possible. But symptoms have a communicative function. Listen to what they are saying to you.
2. After a careful analysis, take action on the body's message. Tailor the remedy to the particular symptom. If possible, choose a non-pharmacological approach. That's what Dixie Koldjeski did. Read on for a great example of self-healing:

> *Several years ago, I realized that I had developed a pattern of splitting headaches in conflict situations in which no kind of resolution occurred. These situations most often happened at work. A favorite expression became: "I am so mad I could spit." After one such expostulation, my husband said, "Why don't you? Maybe you will feel better!" Suddenly I realized that I probably needed to spit out (express) my anger in more productive ways. My strategy for handling anger was a form of self-punishment. I muttered, I simmered, I fumed, and took no purposive action. I eventually faced up to the fact that a psychophysiological response to anger was a very human response—even for a psychiatric/mental health nurse—and had to be dealt with through some kind of intervention. My preference was to use an intervention that was nonpharmacological. My quest took me on a number of discovery experiences until I found one that is effective for me. It has two phases.*

Phase 1: Redirecting Feelings

The first phase is to make myself recognize my anger. This consists of using verbal and body cues that an interaction has aroused anger. At this point, I suggest that those of us involved in the interaction take responsibility for what is happening. Acknowledgment of feelings at this point can open the door to identifying what is preventing movement toward some kind of resolution. I state my position as tactfully as possible and listen to that of others. If communication can be established that acknowledges feelings and areas of conflict, there is a good possibility that interactions will have a successful conclusion. For me, this Phase 1 intervention has been successful in reducing my anger-provoked headaches and making conflictual interactions more collegial and resolvable. But when my Phase 1 intervention does not work, I go to Phase 2.

Phase 2: Mind and Body Engagement

I think of Phase 2 as "using my head for something besides a headache." But before I describe my intervention, I need to digress a moment to explain a situation that was quite significant in helping me to develop it. Bear with me please.

Our home is on a tidal inlet that connects to the ocean. Oysters, clams, and scallops are plentiful, and I have sat many hours watching them survive through the cycles of tides. Mollusks have powerful muscles for attachment, protection, and feeding purposes. Only an hour before and after the tide changes—ebb tide—can they relax their muscles to move around without being at the mercy of the tidal pulls. The message to me was that I needed to create a situation when I had a headache that would allow me to relax and free myself from the pulls of interactions and demands made by others.

This is what I do.

When my Phase 1 intervention is not working—when it becomes apparent that there is no intent by participants to reach a resolution—I accept that . . . temporarily. Next, I find a solitary place. I lie down, put on a Mozart sonata at very low volume, and begin the process of freeing my mind of the persons and circumstances involved in the anger-producing situation. I relax my body and my mind to become like a mollusk—free to give up old ways of doing and thinking and to explore. In my mind, this freeing-up process is analogous to the mollusks' being free from the tidal forces that push them hither, thither, and yon, giving them the freedom to move themselves, find a new attachment, or find new food sources. So I visualize myself as a mollusk to get this state of nirvana, becoming freer and freer of concerns. As I do this, I usually drift into a light slumber for 10 to 15 minutes. When I suddenly awake, I find myself feeling different, free from burden, my headache gone. Now I can think at a lower level of emotionality about the anger-producing situation and consider some new ways of handling it. I go on to identify what to do next and do it.

Well, my strategy works for me. I rarely get headaches anymore. And unlike mollusks which become easy prey to harvesters at ebb tide, I haven't been caught and ended up in a stew—yet!

ANGER'S LINK TO HYPERTENSION AND CORONARY HEART DISEASE

We turn now to cardiovascular sequelae of anger. Anger causes the largest blood pressure increase of any other emotion or mood state— even more than fear (G. Schwartz, Weinberger, & Singer, 1981; J. Schwartz, Warren, & Pickering, 1994). Now that researchers have the capability of using ambulatory blood pressure monitoring, a number of studies have examined workplace anger. Both systolic and diastolic blood pressure are strongly related to angry thoughts and behaviors at work (Durel et al., 1989). Given nurses' reports that their workplaces are rife with hostilities (Brooks et al., 1996; Smith, Droppleman, & Thomas, 1996), it is likely that their blood pressures become elevated many times during a shift. Some of the nurses we interviewed were acutely aware of this. Greg James, when describing an angry incident to our research team, reported, "My blood pressure went to 200. I could feel my hands shaking. I could feel my heart speeding up and my face getting red."

Blood pressure increases are particularly notable during interpersonal conflicts. In one study, blood pressure rose considerably during a discussion of marital problems, attaining a mean of 160/100 mm Hg (Ewart, Taylor, Kraemer, & Agras, 1991). After an angry interaction, it takes quite a while for the pressure to return to normal—as long as 25 minutes in one study (Engebretson, Matthews, & Scheier, 1989). Logically, if you suppress the anger, the physiological arousal will last longer than if you take some action to discharge it. What do most of us do when we get angry at work? We suppress it. Over and over, day after day. Eventually, we could develop hypertension. Prospective studies (Perini,

Muller, & Buhler, 1991) show that suppressed anger accelerates early development of hypertension, although other factors (such as family history of hypertension) are involved as well. This is a good time to point out that no claim is being made here that anger is the sole etiologic agent of the diseases we are focusing on. There is growing recognition that all disease is multifactorial in origin, resulting from a combination of genetic, environmental, and behavioral-emotional factors. Obviously, some of these factors, such as our hereditary predispositions, cannot be modified, but angry thoughts and behaviors can be. One of the basic premises of this book is that emotional habits are *learned*, and therefore they can be *changed*.

Steps Toward Healing

1. Make an assertive response to anger provocation. In a study done by Kathleen Lawler, a colleague at the University of Tennessee, blood pressure levels were monitored while the subjects recalled and described an angry incident. Women who made assertive responses significantly decreased their diastolic blood pressure (Anderson & Lawler, 1994). You'll find complete coverage of assertiveness in Chapter 10.

2. If you can't make an assertive response, find a confidant and get those angry feelings off your chest. Choose wisely, however. You want someone who will simply listen, not offering you advice or fueling more anger by making inflammatory comments. Discussing your anger in this way has clear benefits. In a study of our own, women and men who regularly talked about anger incidents with a confidant had lower systolic and diastolic blood pressures, as well as better general health status (Thomas, 1997a). And in a subsequent study that involved only females, those who suppressed their anger (i.e., scored low on the variable "anger expressed at home") had significantly higher systolic and diastolic blood pressures (Thomas, 1997b).

3. If you can't do either of the first two steps, at least discharge the anger through physical activity. Run, jog, hit a tennis ball. You can combine imagery with any of these. For example, as you run, imagine yourself outrunning the anger, leaving it far behind. As you play tennis, envision a good swat at the person who provoked your anger each time you smash that tennis ball across the net. It's very therapeutic! You can even use household chores to dissipate the anger that built up all day at work. As you empty the garbage, empty your psyche of the workday garbage as well. Regardless of

what happened, it won't do you any good to hold onto that anger all evening. And you need some R&R before you go back to the salt mines tomorrow! So let the anger go.

Now let's take a look at coronary heart disease (CHD). The biological mechanisms by which anger may increase the risk of CHD include discharge of catecholamines, increased myocardial oxygen demand, vasospasm, and increased platelet aggregability. Cardiologists Friedman and Rosenman (1974) considered anger and hostility an important part of the coronary-prone behavior pattern, although it has taken a host of scientific studies over the years to validate just how important it is. The best evidence is from longitudinal studies such as the Western Collaborative Group Study, the Framingham Study, the Tecumseh Study, and the Normative Aging Study, in which initially healthy individuals were enrolled and then followed over a number of years so that researchers could ascertain which predictors proved to be significant in the development of heart disease. The research findings with regard to anger are somewhat different for men and women. We'll start with men.

The Western Collaborative Group Study was the first big study of coronary-prone behavior, dubbed "Type A" by Friedman and Rosenman. The all-male sample included more than 3,000 subjects. After $8\frac{1}{2}$ years Type A men were twice as likely to have symptoms of heart disease than Type B men. Furthermore, the angry, competitive Type A pattern of behavior increased cardiac risk independently of other known risk factors, such as elevated cholesterol, smoking, and high blood pressure. Of the men who died of coronary heart disease during the longitudinal study, 88% were Type As (Rosenman, et al., 1975). I'm sure you remember the rash of media publicity that followed the publication of these findings. Everyone was talking about Type A. But you may not have kept up with the subsequent research literature (unless you're a specialist in cardiac care). In the past two decades, this line of research has taken some interesting twists and turns. Some of the original components of the Type A pattern have turned out to be unrelated to heart disease, but anger and hostility have proved to be key elements.

For men, overtly aggressive, hostile behavior is the most consistent predictor of coronary risk (Hecker, Chesney, Black, & Frautschi, 1989). Hostility is not the same thing as anger; it's a cynical, distrustful mindset. In popular parlance, we might speak of a perpetual chip on one's shoulder. How does hostility relate to anger? Hostile people are highly reactive to events that would not threaten or rile the ordinary person, frequently exploding in outbursts of anger. For example, a hostile person goes ballistic when another driver butts ahead in traffic or a coworker is inefficient or clumsy. While these things are annoying to most of us, the reaction of a hostile person is extreme. In hostile men, anger causes dangerous increases not only in blood pressure but also in stress hormones and testosterone. For these men, expressing the anger outwardly is more strongly associated with cardiovascular hyperresponsivity than having the angry feelings but holding them inside (Suarez & Williams, 1989, 1990; Suarez, Williams, Kuhn, & Schanberg, 1990). In the Normative Aging Study, individuals who had CHD at a 7-year follow-up were those who had admitted back in 1986 that they were hotheaded and sometimes felt like swearing, fighting, or smashing things (Kawachi, Sparrow, Spiro, Vokonas, & Weiss, 1996).

Both hostility and overt anger expression are correlated with atherosclerosis. When we are angry, adrenaline stimulates fat cells, which empty into the bloodstream. If the fat isn't burned, the liver converts it into more cholesterol, which collects in the blood vessels. Over time, the cholesterol forms plaque. Research shows that people with high levels of hostility have more severe blockages of their coronary arteries due to atherosclerotic plaque and more coronary heart disease (Williams et al., 1980). Overt anger expression (e.g., yelling, tantrums) was the critical determinant of coronary artery stenosis severity in a study by Siegman, Dembroski, and Ringel (1987). In cardiac patients whose arteries are already narrowed by plaque, anger causes the vessels to constrict (Boltwood, Taylor, Burke, Grogin, & Giacomini, 1993), reducing left ventricular ejection fraction (Ironson et al., 1992) and producing chest pain (Beaupre, Carney, Freedland, & Eisen, 1994) and even acute myocardial infarction (Mittleman et al., 1995). And the story's not over: Hostility even undermines the benefits of angioplasty, as shown in a study of patients in Baltimore. The risk of restenosis was more than doubled in the patients who scored high on hostility (Goodman, Quigley, Moran, Meilman, & Sherman, 1996).

Although there *are* hostile women—and they are at risk for heart disease like their male counterparts—studies consistently show that hostile, aggressive behavior is much more prevalent in men. This gender difference makes sense to me, because the disease-prone behavior we've been talking about is merely a more extreme version of the competitive "get them before they get you" macho response style that is inculcated in many males from a very early age. Gender role socialization for young boys often includes lessons on how to achieve power with their words and physical strength. Which brings us to the socially approved behavior for the female gender: being "nice" and keeping a lid on our anger.

When it comes to heart health, traditional gender role socialization hasn't served women any better than it has served men. Having to hide or deny a strong emotion like anger produces a number of deleterious consequences. One interesting line of research looks at cardiovascular reactivity when individuals are placed in anger-producing situations. Reactivity is important because it is considered a predictor of coronary heart disease risk. Cardiovascular reactivity experiments commonly employ criticism of the subjects' performance on challenging tasks. The experimenter may say things like "You're still too slow" or "You're obviously not good at doing this; try harder." In one such study of women, the resultant anger was measured as well as the denial of the anger. Subjects scoring high on denial of anger were highly reactive, as indicated by their blood pressures and heart rates (Emerson & Harrison, 1990).

In the well-known Framingham Heart Study, a prospective study of heart disease risk factors, not showing or discussing anger predicted increased incidence of coronary heart disease (Haynes, Feinleib, & Kannel, 1980). I'm sure it doesn't surprise you that the Framingham data also showed that women who work in the human service professions stifle a lot of their anger. Nurses, teachers, and librarians were less likely to show overt anger than housewives or men (Haynes & Feinleib, 1980). In the Tecumseh study, which spanned 18 years, women who suppressed their anger were twice as likely to die of cardiovascular disease (Julius, Harburg, Schork, & DiFrancisco, 1992). In a more recent study, researcher Lynda Powell tracked a group of women who had already had one heart attack for 8 to 10 years to ascertain predictors of subsequent death. The strongest predictor was suppression of emotion (Powell et al., 1993).

To summarize the scientific information in this section of the chapter: Neither scathing attacks nor silent seething promotes healthy hearts. And going around with a negative, hostile outlook or perpetual chip on the shoulder is particularly risky. But coronary-prone behavior *can* be modified, as shown by the success of intervention programs such as the San Francisco Life-Style Heart Trial (Scherwitz & Rugulies, 1992) and the Recurrent Coronary Prevention Project (Powell & Thoreson, 1987). Here are some pointers.

Steps Toward Healing

1. If you have tendencies toward cynical or hostile thoughts, work toward greater tolerance, empathy, and compassion for other people. Most of the people in this world are simply doing the best they can, given their particular life circumstances and coping abilities. Why get bent out of shape when others do not conform to your ideas of efficiency or perfection? Why assume that you know better

than they how they should work, vote, drive, dress, and manage their finances?

2. If you have a tendency to become easily aroused to anger from diverse provocations, learn not to "bite at every hook." Participants in the Recurrent Coronary Prevention Project were taught to imagine themselves as fish (Powell & Thoreson, 1987). Try this imagery yourself: As you swim along each day, numerous "hooks" appear. There are always going to be rude salesclerks and inconsiderate drivers. In the work world of nurses, there are always going to be demanding patients. But you have a choice of whether or not to "bite" at these daily "hooks."

3. Turn down the volume when you express anger verbally. Researcher Aron Siegman and his colleagues conducted experiments in which the subjects talked about anger-arousing events in three different ways: "fast and loud," "slow and soft," or "normally." The researchers found that the highest heart rate and blood pressures occurred when subjects spoke "fast and loud " (Siegman, Anderson, & Berger, 1990). Bolstering my case that new anger habits can be learned, Siegman trained people to talk slowly and softly when angry. The results were quite positive: There was a reduction in the anger itself and in all of the elevated cardiovascular measurements (Siegman & Boyle, 1992).

4. Try the Freeze-Frame technique that is used at the Institute of HeartMath in California to disengage from strong emotional reactions to a situation. The five-step self-management technique involves recognizing your feelings, then shifting the focus away from the disturbed emotion to the physical area around your heart. Then recall a positive emotion such as love or appreciation for someone or something. Feel this feeling. Then, using your intuition, ask your heart what a better response to the situation would be, and listen to what your heart says in answer to the question. Research shows that individuals trained in this technique can use it in real-life stressful situations in the workplace. A transition occurs in heart rate variability waveforms from a noisy wave of large amplitude to a harmonic wave of similar amplitude and then to a smaller amplitude wave (Tiller, McCraty, & Atkinson, 1996).

5. Meditate. A 58-year-old heart patient decided to follow cardiologist Dean Ornish's rigorous low-fat diet and exercise regimen, which has been highly publicized because of its success in actually reversing arterial clogging (Ornish, 1990). However, he could not make such radical changes in his lifestyle in one fell swoop. So he called Ornish and asked him to recommend the single most im-

portant component in the treatment regimen. Dr. Ornish's reply? "Meditate." Give it a try. (We will have more to say about the practice of meditation in Chapter 9.)

ANGER'S LINK TO ADDICTIONS

My colleagues who work in substance abuse treatment are well aware of anger's link to addictions. There is even an acronym—HALT—used by Alcoholics Anonymous to remind its members that they are especially vulnerable to craving a drink when they are Hungry, Angry, Lonely, or Tired. Many of us can identify with this acronym because we too want something to make such feelings go away. Every one of us chooses something to numb our discomfort—perhaps mindless TV watching, compulsive eating, a shopping spree; the addict chooses chemicals. Schaub and Schaub (1997) point out that the early stage of addiction is marked by acceptance of chemicals as a way to change "unsafe feelings." The type of chemical chosen has something to do with the specific feelings the person is trying to assuage. Obviously, sedatives appeal more to the person who is anxious or rageful, while stimulants are attractive to someone who is depressed or shy. In opiate addicts, the most striking emotional pattern is their lifelong difficulty handling anger and rage; with opiates, they finally feel normal and relaxed (Khantzian, cited in Goleman, 1995). In a study of female marijuana users, smoking increased on days when the women experienced anger (Babor, Lex, Mendelson, & Mello, 1984). A nurse in our study who turned to alcohol to numb her rage and anger related:

I can remember as a new grad coming home and needing a couple of stiff drinks every night. You kill yourself all day and then you numb out at night. I could not allow myself to look at the rage and look at the anger.

While an occasional use of a chemical remedy to soothe your anger and tension is not problematic, habitual reliance on a drink or a pill becomes cause for concern. Nurses are an at-risk group for chemical dependency because they have such easy access to powerful mood-altering drugs and are accustomed to thinking of drugs to relieve pain. When Sally Hutchinson studied the process through which nurses became dependent on drugs and/or alcohol, the nurses described both physical and psychological pain. Living itself was painful for them, and they sought to obliterate their pain with chemicals. They used a variety of drugs until they found their drug of choice, the one that "made those horrible feelings go away" or provided "temporary amnesia" (Hutchinson, 1986, p. 198). They justified use of the drug or alcohol to alleviate the pain and help them survive the day. Hutchinson's research documents a tragic trajectory toward self-annihilation. As drug use increased, the nurses withdrew from family and friends. Later on, physical addiction became dominant and normal life became impossible. The nurses took patient medication for their own use, even using while they were on duty. Suicidal ideation and attempts were extremely common. Hutchinson comments: "Ironically, the nurses' attempts at self-care backfired, ultimately bringing more pain than ever" (p. 200).

The facts and figures about the drug problem in our profession are quite disturbing. The incidence of chemical dependency is 50% higher in nurses than in the general population (Kabb, 1984). According to the American Nurses Association, 8% to 10% of nurses have serious problems with drugs or alcohol, which would be around 200,000 of us—and the number may be even higher than that. Studies show that nurse addicts often grew up in chaotic families in which they experienced victimization (Mynatt, 1996). Many had parents who were alcoholic or depressed (Mason, 1995). As adults, these nurses have feelings of distrust, low self-esteem, and anger toward society (O'Quinn-Larson, 1989).

Patterns of nurse drug use vary according to age and gender. Older nurses tend to use more alcohol and prescription drugs, while younger nurses are more likely to use marijuana and cocaine (Tirrell, 1994). Male nurses are more likely than females to be dependent on narcotics (Mason, 1995). Consistent with research on the general population showing that heavy use of one substance is highly correlated with the use of others (Lex, 1991), polydependence is also characteristic of many nurses (Tirrell, 1994). The chemical use of nurses tends to be solitary rather than social (Mason, 1995).

The story of Chuck Mann illustrates many of the dry facts and figures in the preceding paragraphs. Chuck's drug use was so secret that neither his colleagues nor his wife knew about it. He had been working double shifts for months, trying to support his wife and four kids. Says Chuck, "I was the guy you could always call at the last minute and get to come in to work the 11–7 on Saturday night." Sometimes he skimped on a patient's dose of narcotics to obtain a little relief for himself. He'd been sure that, as a nurse, he could control his drug use. But at the time he was fired from his job in a burn unit, his habit was up to about 130 to 140 mg of morphine plus six to eight oxycodone (Percodan) tablets a day (Sandroff, 1982).

Chemical dependency is a complex phenomenon, characterized by a number of physiological abnormalities. The research on alcoholism alone is voluminous, and we cannot examine it here. Most recently, researchers have focused on the association between low serotonin levels and alcohol abuse (Azar, 1997). Given the subsequent media deluge about serotonin, one author facetiously proposed giving alcoholics a "booster shot" of the neurotransmitter, via one of the SSRI (selective serotonin reuptake inhibitor) medications like Prozac, to eliminate their problems. However, no one knows whether low serotonin causes the problems or the problems cause low serotonin. It's too early to pin our hopes on a magic pill. In fact, the proposition—even if facetious—says something about the tendency of so many Americans to rely on a chemical solution rather than taking a closer look at the emotional pain itself.

Alcohol is a dangerous remedy for the emotional pain of nurses, whether male or female. Men are more likely than women to drink and to become heavy drinkers (SAMSHA, 1995). But women progress more rapidly from the onset of drinking to problem drinking and the stages of alcoholism (Orford & Keddie, 1985). The enzyme responsible for the metabolism of alcohol in the stomach does a less thorough job in women (Frezza et al., 1990). A shorter period of drinking produces anemia, ulcers, malnutrition, high blood pressure, and other health consequences for women, as compared to men (Ashley et al., 1977). Women are also more vulnerable to alcohol-induced liver diseases such as cirrhosis (Kilbey & Sobeck, 1988). Another reason for special concern about female nurses is the stigma society attaches to women's drinking, which can be a barrier to getting professional help.

It is interesting—and problematic—that no such stigma is attached to women's taking pills. Women may have to hide their whiskey bottles, but they do not have to hide their tranquilizers, sedatives, and analgesics—especially when the drugs have been medically legitimated by a physician's prescription. Women are more willing than men to report psychological distress to their doctors, and many doctors expect women to need mood-altering medications. Drugs may be offered without careful assessment of a woman's emotional state or exploration of alternative approaches. For as long as I can remember, statistics have consistently shown that twice as many women are given prescriptions for psychotropic medications (Cafferata, Kasper, & Bernstein, 1983). Data from a National Institute on Drug Abuse survey about drug use over the life span revealed that 99% of women age 35 and over who had used tranquilizers, sedatives, or analgesics had been given prescriptions for them (Horton, 1992). Once women receive prescriptions for psychotropic drugs, they tend to continue using them for an extended period (Cooperstock, 1978). Women are more likely than men to misuse and become addicted to prescription drugs (Horton, 1992). Obtaining a prescription is even easier for RNs than for the general population, because a nurse can simply ask a physician with whom she works. The nurses in the study by Hutchinson (1986) said that getting medication from physicians was "a piece of cake."

Even if physicians begin to take a stronger stance against pharmacological remedies for women's psychological pain, many women will still self-medicate with one of the 500,000 over-the-counter (OTC) preparations that require no doctor's order. In a study of our own, midlife women with higher anger symptomatology were high users of both OTCs and alcohol (Grover & Thomas, 1993). Women have a much higher probability of using OTC tranquilizers than men (Bell, 1984). The most frequent user of OTC drugs is a white, middle-class woman (Schuckit, 1989). And of course the "average" nurse, in terms of a statistical profile, is a white, middle-class woman.

If you—or a colleague you care about—are using chemicals to unwind after work or make it through a stressful time, bear in mind that you can become physically addicted accidentally (Hutchinson, 1986). Perhaps you are still telling yourself that you just need the chemicals to get through your divorce. One of the best nurses I ever knew—the epitome of the competent clinician—became an alcoholic after intensifying her drinking during a divorce. What a loss to the profession! Don't let this happen to you. Drug use can interfere with your delivery of safe nursing care and eventually lead to loss of your nursing license. The havoc drugs can wreak in your personal life is immeasurable.

The night Chuck Mann was summarily fired by his supervisor, he walked the darkened streets of Birmingham trying to figure out the easiest way to commit suicide. He did not know how he could go home and tell his wife he'd lost his job. Finally, he dialed the number of a 24-hour crisis hotline and was convinced by the counselor to delay taking his life until morning, when he could be seen at a mental health center. Says Chuck, "Getting off drugs is the hardest thing I ever had to do" (cited in Sandroff, 1982, p. 46). But he was surprised at the support he got when he told his parents, in-laws, neighbors, and friends that he was a recovering addict. Now he counsels other nurse addicts, offering them friendship and hope. If you have a problem with chemicals, there is reason for hope for you too. Current research is demonstrating that the biochemical abnormalities associated with addiction can be reversed through learning. Cognitive therapy and other psychosocial interventions can and do help. But the earlier the intervention, the better the prognosis. Here's how to start down the path to healing.

Steps Toward Healing

1. The first step is to acknowledge that you have a problem with alcohol or drugs. You have a problem if your answer is yes to two or more of the following questions (taken from Fleming & Barry, 1992):

   Have you felt you ought to cut down on your drinking (or drug use)?

   Have people annoyed you by criticizing your drinking (or drug use)?

   Have you felt bad or guilty about your drinking (or drug use)?

   Have you ever had a drink (or used drugs) first thing in the morning to steady your nerves or to get rid of a hangover (or to get the day started)?

   Perhaps you are saying to yourself: "I don't have a problem, I can still respond negatively to these questions." But you may be headed down the road to a more serious problem. Developing psychological dependency is certainly cause for concern. Here are the early signs of psychological dependency:

   Keeping a supply of the substance on hand

   Becoming restless and dissatisfied when the substance is unavailable

   Planning activities around use of the substance

   If you recognize that you are exhibiting these symptoms of psychological dependency, why wait until you are physically addicted to get help? As shown in Hutchinson's research, there's no way to go but down.

2. Become involved in treatment. A good place to begin looking for a facility may be your institution's Employee Assistance Program (EAP). No stigma is attached to seeking help from an EAP, and confidentiality is maintained. Detoxification will be essential. Although alternative modalities such as Outward Bound experiences, art therapy, and meditation are being incorporated into addiction treatment, most professionals still recommend involvement in a 12-step program. In my own clinical experience with chemically dependent patients, I have observed the enormous healing power of Alcoholics Anonymous and Narcotics Anonymous. I believe the power of these programs is derived from their emphasis on spirituality. You must stand humbly before God

(however you understand God) and take a personal inventory. As you complete the first step, you will be asked to give examples of feelings and emotions you have tried to alter with the use of alcohol or other drugs. Later, you will learn how to achieve "natural highs" without substances.

3. Allow others to support you. In AA you will find a community of persons who are trying to "walk their talk" just like you are. Accept the fellowship that is offered you, and let your nurse colleagues support you too. Most states now have organized programs (Peer Assistance or Impaired Nurse programs) that provide confidential, compassionate help. Canada has a program called Project Turnabout (Gaskin, 1986). Contact your state board of nursing or nurses' association for more information. Nurses' AA groups are active in many locales, and if none exists in your area, you may want to start one.

4. Do all that you can to prevent relapse. Appropriate recognition and expression of anger and hurt will help prevent relapse. Danger signs are out-of-proportion anger, blaming, and self-pity. If you do have a relapse, forgive yourself. Realize that you have a chronic disease and, therefore, relapses are to be expected. Recovery is a process. Take heart that thousands of recovering nurses are back on the job. When you have a relapse, climb back on the wagon again. What is important is marshaling courage to renew your commitment to a drug-free life. A drugged existence is a pseudo-life, a living death. You are not fully alive when your emotions are deadened by chemicals. One of our study participants phrased it like this:

> *Drugs are a way of padding the cell, of not meeting your anger head on. And what I mean by padding it, they make you go to sleep and you're not thinking when you're asleep with drugs.*

And now a word about smoking. Let me tell you a little story about student nurses and smoking that still saddens me. I had been invited to another university to give a speech. Although I had been given clear directions regarding how to get to the university, I was not sure exactly where the nursing department was located. I drove around the pleasant, tree-lined campus, reading the names of the buildings. As I rounded a bend, I saw a crowd of young people smoking on the steps outside one particular building. In a flash it occurred to me: "This must be the nursing building!" And so it was. While some individuals acquire the smoking habit before entering nursing school, Elkind (1988) found that there was a trend toward increased consumption during the first year. Interestingly, the students who smoked did not experience greater stress than the nonsmokers, but they felt more anger. How sad to think of a new generation of nurses becoming hooked on cigarettes. Many of my generation were hooked (including me). Shift report often took place in a room thick with smoke. In psychiatric settings, everybody smoked—staff and patients alike. Now clinical agencies are becoming smoke-free, but many nurses still go outside for smoke breaks when they can.

Plenty of nurses are still puffing away: A review of 73 studies on nurses' smoking in 21 countries showed that smoking is still prevalent among both female and male nurses, and in many countries the percentage of nurses who smoke remains higher than that for the general population (Adriaanse, Van Reek, Zandbelt, & Evers, 1991). Female hospital nurses are more likely to smoke than females in similar occupations such as teaching (Ferguson & Small, 1985). Smoking is especially prevalent among hospital nurses who work rotating shifts: In one study, 43.5% of a sample of rotating shift workers smoked (Barak et al., 1996).

Perhaps you have never thought of smoking in connection with anger. But there is a fair amount of research showing that many people acquire the smoking habit in situations of conflict and anger (Theorell & Lind, 1973), use nicotine to regulate their moods (Hughes, 1985), and have difficulty controlling anger and tension when they try to quit smoking. A British researcher found that student nurses who experienced difficulties with staff in their early ward placements were more likely to start smoking (Spencer, 1982). Smoking relapse is associated with anger and loneliness (Macnee, 1991), just as drinking is. In the Women's Anger Study, smoking was more prevalent in unmarried women and in women who admitted to more depressive symptoms (Seabrook, 1993). From my clinical practice as a psychiatric nurse, I became aware of smoking as a coping mechanism long ago. I often observed that just as strong emotion was coming to the surface, a client would light up a cigarette. As the client vigorously puffed, he or she quite effectively created a "smoke screen" that camouflaged the emotion from view. The nicotine gradually produced the relaxation that might have been achieved by talking through the angry feelings.

Nicotine is one of the most toxic and addictive drugs known (Ray & Ksir, 1987). It causes dependence, increased tolerance, and withdrawal symptoms on cessation of use. Some people become severely depressed when they stop smoking, as noted by Christen and Cooper (1979, p. 11): *"At one of our clinics a woman was overheard to say that she mourned more when she quit smoking than she did when her husband died."* Clearly, quitting smoking is not an easy proposition. Studies show that women are more resistant to quitting than men (Stoto, 1986), perhaps because they, more so than men, rely on cigarettes to deal with negative emotion (Biener, 1987). The statistics are grim. Smoking contributes to almost 400,000 deaths per year (Gorman, 1997). Lung cancer has now surpassed breast cancer as the leading cancer killer of women. Yet many nurses have been unable to quit. Knowledge alone is never enough to bring about behavior change, especially when we are speaking of a physiological and psychological addiction. The good news is that it *is* possible to quit. Millions have done so successfully—44 million in the United States. I kicked the habit when I was 27 and caring for two female patients in their 40s—one a nurse, the other a teacher—who were dying of lung cancer. One of them smoked until the end. It made a profound impression on me to see her remove her oxygen, sneak to the bathroom to smoke, and return to bed, gasping for breath, with ghastly cyanosis. I finished my last package of cigarettes and never bought another.

Many people have found a nicotine patch or gum helpful in quitting smoking, although some researchers have concluded that smokers who are angry, tense, and/or depressed may need psychotherapy in addition (Brody, 1994). There are many self-help strategies you can use too. Read on for some good ideas.

Steps Toward Healing

1. There is no right way to quit smoking. You do not have to quit cold turkey. Nor do you have to participate in an organized smoking cessation program. More than 90% of successful quitters do so on their own (Fiore et al., 1990). Explore the various approaches and choose the one that is right for you.

2. Once you have made the decision to quit, get rid of all smoking materials. Remove ashtrays, lighters, and other smoking paraphernalia from your home. Freshen your environment by cleaning the draperies and carpets and changing furnace filters.

3. Make a public commitment to your family and colleagues and ask for their support. Perhaps you can persuade your spouse or a friend to quit smoking with you. Warn your support persons that you will probably be irritable and unpleasant during nicotine withdrawal.

4. If you fear weight gain, be aware that the average weight gain after smoking cessation is only 5 pounds (U.S. Department of Health and Human Services, 1990a).

5. Find a substitute activity (crunching ice, chewing gum, eating fruit, sipping fluids). When I quit smoking, I missed cigarettes the most

after meals. My substitute was a cup of coffee. (If you need to avoid caffeine, make it decaf.)
6. Don't try to quit smoking until you've learned effective ways of managing your anger and other negative emotions. Relaxation and imagery are helpful to many people.

While some nurses would not think of smoking or drinking, they do indulge in another kind of drug to medicate emotional pain: food. A pain-killing peptide, CCK, is released in the gut after a meal, creating a feeling of well-being (Hall, 1989). Some of the participants in the Women's Anger Study were keenly aware that they used food as a drug:

Food is such a wonderful drug. It's so easily accessible. Nobody's ever gonna bust me for havin' a burger and fries in the car.

When I'm angry, I want to eat. Some people's stomachs close up. Mine says, "Feed me, feed me."

Fat is really my drug of choice. . . . I have eaten cheese, particularly, a lot . . . escapades with mayonnaise . . . when used as a drug it's just to numb my feelings.

As with an occasional beer or margarita, an occasional food fix for anger or stress may not be a problem. But 100 extra calories a day results in 10 extra pounds a year, and most "mood foods" have far more than 100 calories. Once you've started munching, it is very difficult to stop. Weight can become a very "weighty" problem, especially for women. Women eat more in response to mood states than men do (Forster & Jeffery, 1986). Across all age groups, women are more obese than men. I found no studies on obesity in male nurses, but a study that compared female nurses to women in the general population found a higher percentage of the nurses to be overweight (Pratt, Overfield, & Hilton, 1994).

Obese women are stigmatized in our society because they do not conform to the culturally approved lean and leggy look. Thus, the longing to be slimmer sends millions of us to weight loss programs, where we outnumber men 9 to 1 (Bennett, 1991). Many of us become angry at ourselves for food excesses and inability to shed the pounds, which leads us back to anger (yes, it's a vicious cycle, as shown in the research conducted by my colleagues Sheryl Russell and Barbara Shirk in 1993).

We know from the scientific literature that obesity is partly the result of genetics, but there are many other contributing factors—among them anger and hostility. Susie Orbach (1978) was one of the first authors to take a feminist stance, alleging that women's subordinate role to fathers, husbands, or bosses forced them to stuff their anger—and literally stuff their mouths full of food—rather than express anger or disagreement. More recently, Kim Chernin (1985) and Judi Hollis (1994) have advanced the notion that women's need to sedate their anger with food can be traced back to the troubled relationship between mothers and daughters. Hollis, founder of the nation's first eating disorders hospital unit, explicitly linked overweight and anger in the title of her book *Fat and Furious: Women and Food Obsession.*

Whether or not you view fat as a feminist issue, like Orbach does, or find the arguments of Chernin and Hollis compelling, you can attest from your own experience that certain fattening foods do soothe negative moods. Women tend to prefer fat-sugar combinations like chocolate, ice cream, and cake for their mood foods, whereas men like fat-protein or fat-salt mixtures such as steak, pizza, and french fries (Levey, 1994). The idea of food being used to deal with painful emotions precedes Susie Orbach by centuries. In fact, there are references in the Talmud to the connection between negative mood states and weight (Siegman, 1994). As I reviewed the literature, I came across a fascinating 1893 story of a nursing teacher at Johns Hopkins who advocated a cure for melancholia (depressive illness) called "stuffing"—which meant giving the patient as much food as he or she could eat (Steingarten, 1994).

Several recent studies document a link of hostility and anger with overeating and/or obesity. One study found that highly hostile individuals (whether black or white, male or female) consumed a significantly greater number of calories per day than persons who were not very hostile. Highly hostile black men ingested 628 more calories, and black women 490 more calories, than their less hostile counterparts; hostile white men admitted 594 more calories and white women 295 more calories per day (Scherwitz & Rugulies, 1992). In a study of college students, covert hostility was strongly related to compulsive eating (Kagan & Squires, 1984). In the Women's Anger Study, we found higher obesity in women who reported greater use of anger suppression or anger ventilation that was done in an attacking, blaming way (Russell & Shirk, 1993). Research also shows that anger contributes to relapses from diets (Grilo, Shiffman, & Wing, 1989). In the words of one of our study participants, it is easy to "fall off the wagon" and resort to food for solace when upset:

What the hell; I might as well eat. They don't like me, I didn't get the job, whatever.

Food binges are described with remarkable similarity to episodes of heavy drinking or drug use:

> *I can eat anything to excess. I can binge on carrots; I really can. If I were to eliminate all the foods that I can use for medicating myself, I guess I'd be left with garlic and a leaf of rhubarb or something; mango chutney maybe.*

> *One dose of sugar could lead to another and another and another. It's an addiction. Maybe someday I can sit down and have a piece of chocolate and say, "Wasn't that good?" and that's enough, but now I'd eat it and want more.*

Do these quotes from our data sound like things that you might say? If so, it's time to consider alternatives to eating when emotionally upset. In focus groups conducted by members of our research team (Russell & Shirk, 1993), some excellent ideas were shared. Amanda has learned not to isolate herself when she is angry or hurt:

> *I have certain things I do now that I wouldn't have done before. Before I would have isolated myself. I might not have even told anybody I was upset, or what was wrong. Now I make myself tell somebody what's going on: "I'm really mad about this" or "I was so hurt when somebody said this." Just not isolate, not keep the feelings inside; let 'em out, get 'em out. Just telling someone helps me, calling up a friend. . . . It's getting out of myself, not keeping feelings inside and then eating them, eating my feelings.*

Here are some other recommendations to help you break the anger-food chain.

Steps Toward Healing

1. Keep a journal to document emotionally induced eating. Analyze each anger incident and make a plan to either resolve the issue or react differently to it in the future.
2. Begin to explore ways to reduce anger arousal without resorting to food. For example, use imagery to transport yourself to a peaceful scene where nothing can bother you.
3. Engage in a physical activity to discharge anger—exercise, gardening, painting, pottery, or other crafts—something completely incompatible with eating.
4. If you must do something oral, try crunching on raw carrots or cauliflower or sip a cool caffeine-free beverage.

5. If you need to diet, don't try a fad or "miracle" plan. Take a sensible approach based on the pyramid food guide (largely whole-grain breads and cereals, fruits, and vegetables). You'll be getting high fiber, which is filling and reduces the need to eat excessive amounts of food to have that feeling of satiation.

A final word about dieting. There is a vociferous antidieting movement in this country. Its principal assertion is that all diets fail. Certainly, the harmful effects of yo-yo dieting are well known. While I do not want to contribute to guilt about weight—since that's rampant already—I do recommend taking a good look at emotionally motivated eating and developing healthy alternatives. Some weight loss may actually follow, even if you have not been "on a diet." Even modest weight loss (of 15 to 30 pounds) produces beneficial changes in blood sugar, insulin, triglycerides, and HDL cholesterol (Dattilo & Kris-Etherton, 1992; Goldstein, 1991; Wing et al., 1987). My position on dieting is that each person must make a careful evaluation in consultation with his or her health care provider.

ANGER'S LINK TO CANCER

Finally, we consider anger's link to cancer. Like so many other diseases, cancer is caused by a combination of factors, including chemical carcinogens and behaviors such as smoking. The emotion of anger is only one of these many factors, and we do not want to overemphasize its importance. But a host of empirical evidence has been accumulating, and we need to review it. One of the earliest prospective studies was conducted by Caroline Thomas and her associates at Johns Hopkins. In 1946, she set out to find an answer to this question: Are specific psychological patterns in youth predictive of future disease and death? Thomas gave medical students at Johns Hopkins various questionnaires and tests such as the Rorschach (inkblot) test. Over the years, when the study participants became ill or died, Thomas and her coworkers categorized the deaths. Striking psychological similarities were found among individuals with the same disease. The outstanding characteristics of the cancer group included low scores on closeness to parents, nervous tension, depression, anxiety, and anger. When compared to groups who had hypertension, heart attack, mental illness, or suicide, the cancer group had the lowest scores of all groups on anger, anxiety, and depression (C. B. Thomas, 1988). The meaning of these findings will become clearer as we consider other research and delve more deeply into what some researchers call the "antiemotionality" of the cancer-prone personality.

Another prospective study, conducted in Yugoslavia, involved initial assessment of anger, depression, anxiety, and a number of other aspects of emotionality. At a 10-year follow-up, the researchers had a 78% success rate in prediction of cancer incidence based on characteristics such as antiemotionality and need for harmony. The incidence of cancer was 40 times greater among individuals who behaved in a rational, unemotional way (Grossarth-Maticek, Bastiaans, & Kanazir, 1985).

Perhaps the best known of the contemporary researchers is Lydia Temoshok, who uses the term *Type C behavior pattern* to describe a set of emotional and behavioral characteristics very similar to those identified in the previous studies. She considers the core factor of the cancer-prone pattern to be nonexpression of emotion. How did she come to this conclusion? From 1978 to 1988 Temoshok studied patients with melanoma. The physicians in the melanoma clinic at the University of California, San Francisco, had asked for her help to study a syndrome of "flat" emotionality that they were observing in the melanoma patients who had the thickest tumors. Temoshok spent hours talking to these patients before she designed her formal studies, noting that these patients were incredibly nice and focused not on their own problems but on pleasing their spouses, parents, and others in their network of relationships. They never expressed anger and only on rare occasions did they express fear or sadness (Temoshok, 1985; Temoshok & Dreher, 1992; 1993).

Steven Greer and his colleagues in London have conducted several studies of women with breast cancer. In Greer's first study, the only attribute that successfully distinguished between benign and malignant breast disease was the way in which women handled their emotions—particularly anger. Both extreme suppressors (those who had not openly shown anger more than once or twice in their lives) and extreme expressors (those who had frequent temper outbursts) had higher rates of diagnosed breast cancer than women with more moderate or "normal" emotional behavior. Among the cancer patients, there were more anger suppressors than exploders (Greer & Morris, 1975; Morris, Greer, Pettingale, & Watson, 1981). In a later study by Greer's research team, breast cancer patients and disease-free women watched stressful videotapes while their physiological reactions were continuously monitored. The cancer patients became more anxious and emotional watching the films than the control group, but they tried to hide their angry reactions and anxiety. However, the researchers were able to detect the discrepancy between the women's heightened physiological arousal and their public facade of emotional control (Watson, Pettingale, & Greer, 1984).

Here is one final piece of research, looking at a different type of cancer: colorectal. Suppressed anger has been identified as a characteristic of patients with colorectal cancer in a study comparing over 600 confirmed cancer cases with cancer-free individuals of the same age and sex. The colorectal cancer patients were found to have experienced significant childhood loss and unhappiness, and their adult personalities were consistent with the Type C profile of the "nice" person who seeks to avoid conflict and keep negative emotions inside (Kune, Kune, Watson, & Bahnson, 1991).

The childhood loss and unhappiness uncovered in this study brings us to another very important point: Many persons with cancer-prone characteristics developed their tendency to keep feelings under wraps as a defense mechanism during earlier life experiences of loss, stress, and trauma. Some had abusive or alcoholic parents, so they learned at an early age: "Don't tell anyone how you feel." What served them well as a survival strategy during childhood pain became dysfunctional—even life-threatening—in adulthood. A woman with lymphoma told of the green shoes her mother had given her, a gift symbolizing the psychological entrapment that she felt contributed to her cancer:

> I had very few clothes as a child, usually just hand-me-downs [from my older brothers and sisters.] My mother would go off on extravagant shopping excursions, but only for herself. Then one day, she came home with something for me! It was a wonderful-looking pair of green suede shoes, with laces and everything. Unfortunately, they were the wrong size, way too small. Still, I never said a word, because I knew [that] if I told her she would just yell at me, or else take them back and not get me any others. So I wore the green shoes, even though every step felt like it was killing me. (Barasch, 1994, p. 311)

Metaphorically, this woman had worn her green shoes until the day she got cancer. She had continually squeezed herself into emotionally cramped adult relationships and thwarted her most creative impulses. Walking in the ill-fitting green shoes was indeed killing her. But neither this woman nor any other cancer victims should be blamed for bringing their disease upon themselves. It is tragic that 41% of breast cancer patients blamed themselves for developing cancer in one recent study (cited in Trafford, 1997). Cancer prone persons do not consciously choose to be the way they are.

Although the biological explanation for the connection of emotional suppression and cancer has not been definitively established, Keith Block, medical director of a cancer institute in Chicago, proposes that habitual suppression of negative emotions such as anger results in oversecretion of opioid peptides. The brain is trying to relieve the emotional pain in the same way that it would combat physical pain. Subsequently, the excess of opioid peptides suppresses the tumor-fighting activity of natural killer cells. This immunosuppression can result in tumor development (Block, 1997).

Self-Assessment

Do you have a Type C personality? Assess yourself on the following characteristics identified by Lydia Temoshok:

Inability to express emotions like anger
Focus on pleasing others
Avoidance of conflict
Appeasing, unassertive manner

Steps Toward Healing

1. If you have characteristics of the cancer-prone personality, embark on a journey of self-discovery through counseling. Take heart that even patients with diagnosed lesions can successfully change Type C behavior. Author Alice Epstein, diagnosed with inoperable cancer but currently alive and whole, has written a book about "reversing" her cancer-prone personality. All of her life she had inhibited anger and sacrificed her own needs to please others; she once got the highest score possible on a test of nonexpression of hostility. Through therapy, she vented all the pent-up emotion: "I was able to rid myself of feelings that I had experienced over a lifetime in a matter of months and sometimes weeks" (Epstein, 1989, p. 201).

   The most dramatic empirical evidence is the success of psychiatrist David Spiegel's group therapy, which has received national media attention. When Spiegel began his therapy group for patients with metastatic breast cancer, his main impetus was to minimize their suffering and enhance the quality of their lives. He quickly found that most of the group time was spent discussing strong negative emotions such as fear and anger that needed to be expressed. The group provided support and encouragement for the expression of these feelings. At a 10-year follow-up, Spiegel found that the women in therapy lived almost twice as long as those who had been assigned to a control group receiving routine medical care. Survival rates improved in direct proportion to the number of group sessions the women attended (Spiegel, Bloom, Kraemer, & Gottheil, 1989).

2. If you are presently battling cancer, research shows that anger can be an antidote to feelings of helplessness and a sparkplug to the immune system. A study by Derogatis and his colleagues (1979) showed that women who openly expressed anger about having cancer had higher rates of survival than those who expressed little or no anger. Lydia Temoshok found that cancer patients who were able to express anger and other emotions had more cancer-killing lymphocytes at their tumor sites. Physician Steven Greer (1990) encouraged his breast cancer patients to mobilize their "fighting spirit," and at 15-year follow-up, the ones with fighting spirit were more likely to be alive.

We have touched on only some of the many health conditions in which mismanaged anger is implicated. If I were writing an exhaustive review of the literature, I would go on to tell you about the research evidence that links anger to chronic pain, rheumatoid arthritis, and many other conditions. But my purpose in writing this book is not to cover all the factual information that is out there. In fact, the literature is burgeoning so rapidly that I can hardly keep up with it. Each new study reinforces my conviction that we must learn—and teach our patients—better ways to manage anger. I hope I have heightened your awareness that what you do with your anger can have important consequences for your health. But we need to move on to strategies for reining in anger that's gone out of control. One of the most important strategies for doing so is learning to distinguish between anger that is rational and anger that is irrational. That is our next topic.

3

Differentiating Between Rational and Irrational Anger

Much of nurses' anger is quite rational. Their emotional response to disrespectful treatment, blaming, and scapegoating is understandable. As you were reading the stories in Chapter 1, I'm sure you could feel your own anger rising in empathic resonance with your colleagues. But not all nurses' anger is rational. As we interviewed RNs, we heard a lot of "oughts" and "shoulds," indicating unrealistic expectations of patients, management, and themselves. Before you can manage anger effectively, you must learn to differentiate between that which is rational and that which is irrational. To borrow a portion of the Serenity Prayer, you need "the wisdom to know the difference." Let's begin this discussion by examining the definition of anger:

Anger is a strong, uncomfortable, emotional response to a provocation that is unwanted and incongruent with one's values, rights, or beliefs.

Notice that the first major element of the definition is that the angry person is responding to something that he or she did not want to happen. For example, my ire can be aroused when I receive unwanted advice "for my own good" or unwanted telephone solicitation for aluminum siding during dinner. Or perhaps I am told to work on an assignment with someone with whom I don't want to work. If my desires, wishes, and preferences remain flexible, they are not necessarily irrational. I can conclude that the annoyances of unwanted advice and telemarketers are relatively minor and not worth stewing about. I can view the work assignment as tolerable, even if it is not what I would prefer. Unfortunately, humans have a tendency to escalate their wants and desires into dogmatic musts about the self, others, and the world/life conditions (Dryden, 1990). This tendency leads to irrational conclusions and negative behavioral consequences. I'll have more to say about this tendency a bit later in the chapter.

The next element of my anger definition emphasizes that the anger-producing situation or incident was incongruent with values, rights, or beliefs. In the pages of this book, you have already seen many examples of nurses' anger in response to provocations that offend their values. A lot of what is happening in the health care delivery system offends our values, because we value patients more so than the obscene profits some health care organizations are making. It sure makes me angry that the hospital industry has enjoyed hefty profits for the past 7 or 8 years while claiming that "health care reform" is mandating reduction in RN staffing. This isn't true, and we know it isn't.

Strong anger on behalf of patients was expressed by many nurses who participated in our studies. This anger on behalf of patients is rational and a sparkplug for advocacy measures. It is anger driven by the humanistic-altruistic value system that is the basis of nursing as a science of caring (Watson, 1985). Linda Harvey became quite emotional as she recounted an incident that occurred when she was working the evening shift on a surgical unit and went to get an elderly patient to sign the permit for a scheduled mastectomy. Finding that the patient was barely literate, Linda read the permit to her and her daughter. But the patient still did not comprehend that removal of her breast was planned; she insisted, "They're going to remove the lump. I don't want my breast removed." Linda called the physician, relating to him, "She understood that she's having a lumpectomy, and that's the only thing she wants." The doctor said, "No, she's going to have a mastectomy. You must have said something to confuse her. Go back and get the permit signed." Linda refused to do so, and here's the rest of the story:

> When I left that night I explained to the oncoming shift that the surgery was going to have to be canceled, or else they were going to have to make sure they were only removing the lump. The next night when I came back to work, the patient had had a mastectomy. The resident had talked to her and she had signed the permit. It was so upsetting. She was a vulnerable person. She was not educated. It was, like you can dupe her because she doesn't understand. There are many times that you are speaking on behalf of the patient: "I said I wanted the lump removed; I didn't say I wanted the

breast removed." So in a sense you're speaking for that person. Being an advocate, to me, encompasses everything.

Ann Smith is a staff nurse in labor and delivery. She tells of a doctor who came in and began fussing at Ann's laboring patient because "she wasn't trying hard enough." Ann relates:

I told the doctor he couldn't talk to her that way . . . I took action. I wrote him up and then I went to his partner and let his partner know what happened. . . . The doctor that I had the confrontation with has been very nice to me. I've not had any more problems with him. He's been very good to my patients. I feel sure something was said to him.

On another occasion, Ann was caring for a young Medicaid patient, and a doctor told her that "Medicaid patients can't get an epidural." Ann asked him repeatedly about the epidural, but he continued to say no. Thoroughly incensed, Ann again acted on behalf of her patient. Whether or not you approve of the tactic she chose, she got results:

I took him outside the door and I said, "Okay, I want you to stand right there. Now, you've got a teenage daughter at home, and I want you to imagine that that's your daughter in that bed. Every time we hear my patient scream when she hurts I'm going to kick you in the shin. I want you to pretend that's your daughter, and me kicking you in the shin is going to be your heart hurting because it's your daughter that the doctor won't give the epidural to." My patient got the epidural and I've never had to deal with it again with that particular doctor.

Let's turn from discussion of values to rights. Recall that my definition of anger also emphasizes violation of our rights as human beings. Applying this element of the definition to nursing, I assert that the nurse has a right to a reasonable workload, respectful treatment from other members of the health care team, and a clearly specified mechanism for resolution of grievances. A "Nurses' Bill of Rights" compiled by Sonja Herman (1978) includes the right to question, challenge, or state opinions, to make decisions about nursing care, to make a mistake, to change one's mind, to say no, to have in writing what is expected at work, and to ask for changes in the system. Instead, the nurses in our study (and studies by others) speak of impossible assignments, sex discrimination, and powerlessness to affect changes in the system. When nurses become angry because situations and events are incongruent with their rights, I believe that their anger is rational and justifiable. Something is wrong and needs to be corrected. In such cases, the emotion of anger should be considered a *gift*.

THE GIFT OF ANGER

The gift of anger should be claimed—and used wisely. It provides strong momentum for activism. As you feel the anger building in your mind and body, realize that you can use its energy in any way you wish. Feel its power. Imagine it propelling you forward to act. Perhaps you must confront someone who is taking advantage of you or failing to do their share of the work. Perhaps you must challenge workplace discrimination or ill-conceived policies. Anger can empower you to do this. Philosopher Robert Solomon (1976) says that anger helps us to "change the world and change ourselves . . . to ask "What will I do now?"

For physician Rachel Naomi Remen, the force of her anger proved to be life-affirming. She became ill at the age of 15 with Crohn's disease. Anger has played different roles during her 35 years with this disease, but she is convinced that it is far healthier than apathy, hopelessness, and resignation:

> *Anger was my way of refusing to accept invalidhood. . . . When I was 15 and I first became ill, I felt an anger that seemed bottomless and lasted for four or five years. I actually hated well people because I felt hopelessly separated from them.*
>
> *I can remember the very moment that I changed. I was walking on a beach thinking how exhausted I was and how I could not go on, and suddenly I had the experience of being filled with a familiar rage. But this time I experienced the* vitality *of my anger: the life energy that had somehow become caught in the form of anger. At that point I recognized it for what it really was. It was my will to live and to resist distortion, and I no longer needed to be angry to experience it. (Remen, 1996, p. 25)*

Emotions evolved for their adaptive value in dealing with fundamental life tasks and predicaments (Ekman, 1994). They are important sources of information about self-identity and personal needs and the actions that are necessary to fulfill those needs (Dafter, 1996). The word *emotion* comes from the Latin *exmovere*, meaning "to move out, to have the experience of being moved." When deeply moved by feelings, we have an altered perspective and behave differently as well. Anger jolts us out of passivity and stimulates us to become movers and shakers. One woman we interviewed spoke of the "buzz" that anger gave her, enabling her to assert herself more emphatically: *"I felt a real buzz. I felt, you know, like 'I'm not going to be treated this way.' I felt strong. I felt like someone was listening to me. . . . I felt in control."* Another woman valued her anger for two reasons: It alerted her, and it energized her to take action on her behalf. She noted, *"My anger makes me find solutions. Whenever I feel angry I try to say, 'Okay, this is an emotion that's alerting me that there is a problem here.' My anger lets me know it's time to take care of something."* Similarly, a nurse saw her anger as "a red flag": *"I see it as a red flag that says, 'Something just happened here—you were violated.' If I acknowledge my anger instead of trying to stuff it, I can identify solutions."*

I like the symbolism of the red flag. It's a symbol with universal meaning: STOP. There is danger. Do not continue on this road. Find an alternate route. Mobilizing anger can be the first step in personal liberation when your course is fraught with danger. There are times in each person's life when a new direction must be taken, a new future constructed, or the self is in danger of extinction. Perhaps you are in a relationship in which you are smothered. Therapist Harriet Lerner (1985, p. 31) reminds us that perpetual anger at someone is an extremely useful clue: "If we are chronically angry or bitter in a particular relationship, that may be a message to clarify and strengthen the 'I' a bit more." No relationship is healthy if one self swamps the other. Anger can be the impetus for breaking free from such a relationship— or from a joyless work role that offers no opportunity for continued growth and advancement. Let me tell you a story. There was an elephant who was staked to the ground with a chain. As a baby, no matter how hard she struggled, she couldn't break free. Now, as an adult, the elephant is big enough and strong enough to gain her freedom. But she doesn't bother to try. Many people in miserable situations are like the elephant. They view their conditions as inevitable: "This is the way things are." Have you, like the elephant, stopped trying? Anger can give you the power to break that chain.

Not long ago, I was admiring a huge, vibrant painting of a single flower in the National Museum of Women in the Arts. No one can paint flowers like Georgia O'Keeffe! Posted beside her glorious painting were some words the artist uttered in 1923: "One day seven years ago I found myself saying to myself: 'I can't live where I want to, I can't go where I want to, I can't do what I want to do, I can't even say what I want to.' . . . I decided I was a very stupid fool not to at least PAINT as I wanted to." And so she boldly began to paint differently from the other artists of the time. The world had never seen anyone paint like she painted. Critics snarled, but Georgia continued to paint as she wanted to. Anger had unleashed her unique and formidable talent, for which all of us can be grateful.

Anger can also unleash moral or righteous anger. If it weren't for righteous anger, many of us would never become involved in social justice projects. It is when we get "good and angry" that we join with others in efforts to save the wilderness, build homes for the homeless, or fight crime in our neighborhoods. I often think about a particular organization, Mothers Against Drunk Driving. Many of the members of this organization have lost a child to a drunken driver. As a mother, I can think of nothing that would produce more grief and rage. These women could choose to remain, like their acronym, MADD, but instead their anger is used constructively to work for better legislation and educate drivers. Similarly, RNs form coalitions to lobby for more enlightened public policy. Development of the document, "Nursing's Agenda for Health Care Reform" (American Nurses Publishing, 1993) is an excellent example. Irate at the large number of Americans with no access to health care and the inadequate, patchwork approaches to health care reform, more than 60 nursing organizations united to write this stirring call for a basic core of services for all people.

Perhaps you have never thought of anger as a gift. Because of its pejorative connotations in our society, many people view anger as pathological or bad, in fact a sin. One of the members of our research team was told from the pulpit that "anger is only a *d* away from *d*anger." Her minister may have confused anger with aggression. There is considerable confusion about the terms *anger, hostility, aggression,* and *violence.* Bear with me for a minute while I define these terms. In the previous chapter, you learned about *hostility,* that mental attitude of antagonism toward the world and the other people in it. *Aggression* involves an actual or impending physical or verbal attack on someone, and *violence* is an unjust, forceful assault that inflicts injury. But ordinary anger is not hostile, aggressive, or violent, and it is not a sin. The research of James Averill (1983) showed that physical aggression during anger is relatively rare in a normal, nonclinical population, occurring in only 10% of angry episodes. What most of us experience in everyday life is anger, a natural and healthy response to a provocation. Anger pertains to events of greater significance than minor irritations or mere annoyances, but it is less enduring and mean-spirited than hostility, and less destructive than aggression or violence (Thomas, 1995).

I am indebted to Carroll Saussy (1995), a professor of pastoral care and counseling, for her insightful "theology of anger." Her exploration refutes the old notion that displaying anger is un-Christian. She carefully examines the Bible's teaching on anger, pointing out that there is a lot of anger in both the Hebrew Bible and the New Testament. Although there are warnings about anger in some passages ("He that is slow to anger is better than the mighty;" "Anger resteth in the bosom of fools"), God gets angry, Jesus gets angry, and anger is an important component of the human lives that are presented in these texts. Anger can be holy, according to Saussy:

> . . . *holy anger [is] a response to the experience of being ignored, injured, trivialized, or rejected, as well as an empathic response aroused by witnessing someone else being ignored, injured, trivialized, or rejected. (1995, p. 115)*

SINFUL ANGER

There *is* sinful anger, defined by Saussy as "a vengeful, hostile, sometimes explosive reaction [that] aims to injure persons or institutions and tears at the fabric of society by destroying relationships" (1995, p. 115). Sinful anger—which should really be called aggression or violence rather than anger—is attributed to "brokenhearted" persons who have not been respected or loved sufficiently. The etiology of their broken hearts can be dysfunctional family backgrounds, abuse, and/or poverty. The violent acts are attempts to overcome perceived worthlessness and helplessness (Rothenberg, 1973). Nurses see the horrifying consequences in the bruises of battered women, the broken limbs of children, the gunshots and knife wounds that are routine Saturday night fare in the emergency departments of every metropolitan hospital. Often, the destructive anger is taken out on the next generation, perpetuating the brokenheartedness.

I will never forget a boy of about 11 or 12 whom I cared for in the ICU. His father had literally stomped him with heavy boots, along with delivering many blows with his fists. The bootprints, still visible days after his admission, went deep into his flesh. One day his father, a slightly built man in baggy overalls, came into the ICU during the visiting period. I asked him what the boy had done to provoke his anger. It seems the boy had not done his chores properly. I was stunned and sickened by the father's disproportionate reaction. We've all had children who failed to do their chores properly from time to time. But the perpetrators of violent acts such as this never learned healthy ways to manage their angry feelings.

While it is beyond the scope of this book to delve more deeply into the topic of violence, I do believe that all of us must begin to work toward solutions. Violence in America is an ever-growing social problem. Each new set of statistics is more alarming, particularly with regard to the propensity of our young people to settle their disputes with fists and guns. According to Justice Department statistics, between 1988 and 1992 there was a 68% increase in the number of juveniles charged with murder, aggravated assault, robbery, and forcible rape, with aggravated assault up 80% (cited in Goleman, 1995). Although the problem of violence may seem so immense that no individual action can make a dent in it, learning to manage our own anger is a place to start. After we nurses have acquired some skills, we need to teach them to our patients at every opportunity. Psychoeducational programs in both inpatient and outpatient settings could be presented by nurses. Individuals who know no outlet for anger but smashing and beating must learn to put words to their feelings. A 1996 study showed that psychiatric patients who had a hard time verbalizing anger were more likely to release it in the form of violent assaults on staff. Nonviolent patients more often discussed their angry feelings appropriately (Lanza, Kayne, Pattison, Hicks, & Islam, 1996).

Learning to talk about feelings is not enough, of course. Before they will halt their aggressive actions, violent individuals must begin to encounter penalties for their behavior. As we all know, behavior is repeated when it is rewarded. The person who bullies another and gets away with it is surely likely to remain a bully. A disturbing study of juvenile offenders shows that the negative consequences of a violent solution never cross their mind (Slaby & Guerra, 1988). They held beliefs such as "It's okay to hit someone if you just go crazy from anger" and "People who get beaten up badly don't really suffer that much." One of my pet soapbox topics is the glamorized violence on television. The National Television Violence Study revealed that 58% of TV programs contained violence, and three-fourths of violent scenes on TV contained no remorse, criticism, or penalties for violence (Seppa, 1997). I am particularly concerned about impressionable children who have difficulty distinguishing between fantasy and reality. Forty percent of violent incidents on television are initiated by characters that are attractive role models for children (Seppa, 1997). While some argue that violent television programs or movies provide harmless entertainment, I believe otherwise.

Certainly, many of the individuals whom Saussy calls "brokenhearted" need far more than acquisition of coping skills such as talking about their feelings or penalties for aggressive behavior. Some have such severe psychopathology, dating back to abandonment, unmet needs, and abuse in infancy, that intensive treatment will be necessary. They have no trust in other people, little or no impulse control, and no empathy for the suffering of those whom they hurt in the heat of anger. Much work with a trusted therapist will be needed for learning what they missed, as well as developing more normal patterns of response to replace their dysfunctional ones. There is some basis for hope. There are new treatments for aggressive and delinquent children that are achieving successful outcomes (DeAngelis, 1997; Wahler, Cartor, Fleischman, & Lambert, 1993). Additionally, therapists who conduct anger management groups for adults in Veterans Affairs facilities across the country are finding that traumatized adults can learn to control aggression (Gerlock, 1994; Novaco, 1996).

Gerlock (1994), a nurse therapist, led a series of six different 8-week classes with groups of 6 to 12 veterans, most of whom were Vietnam veterans with a diagnosis of posttraumatic stress disorder from their deeply disturbing war experiences. These men had high levels of out-of-control anger and rage on entry into Gerlock's classes. The goals of the treatment were to reduce the level of anger and to promote constructive management of it. Participants were encouraged to take responsibility for their anger behaviors, rather than externalizing blame. As the weeks of treatment went on, Gerlock learned that a large number of the men had been victims of childhood trauma—sexual exploitation, physical violence, witnessing domestic violence—prior to the trauma of their military service in a war zone. Despite the severe trauma that these men had endured, they responded positively to the anger management intervention. There was a statistically significant decrease in their scores on a widely used anger measure that was given at the first and the last classes. One Vietnam combat veteran summed up his learning from treatment as follows: *"I thought I had control because people were afraid of me . . . people feared what I might do. That was a delusion . . . with the anger, I didn't really have control over myself"* (Young, 1996, p. 57). As this veteran now understands, control of emotional behavior is a critical skill to master. Without such control, Vietnam veterans—and you and I—cannot successfully live and work in harmony with others.

EMOTIONAL INTELLIGENCE

I am encouraged that so much attention is now being devoted to "emotional literacy" and "emotional intelligence" in the popular press. Daniel Goleman's book *Emotional Intelligence* (1995) snagged the cover of *Time* and started a national discussion of "EQ." Drawing on the scholarly work of Peter Salovey and John Mayer, Goleman contends that emotional intelligence—the regulation of emotion in a way that enhances living—may be more crucial to personal and professional success than IQ, academic achievement, or acquisition of specific job skills. The cornerstone of EQ is awareness of your own feelings, because with awareness you can learn to exercise self-control and select appropriate coping mechanisms. Goleman recommends, as I have in the previous chapter, tuning in to somatic markers of emotion, our gut feelings. Basic skills include identifying and labeling feelings correctly and knowing the difference between feelings and actions. EQ also involves skills in interpreting social cues, understanding the perspectives of other people, and managing moods effectively.

Most of us had no classes in school to help us develop emotional competence; all of our schooling was focused on acquiring information and technical skills. I was pleased to learn that emotional literacy programs, such as New Haven's Social Competence Program and New York City's Resolving Conflict Creatively Program, are now under way in some schools. Many of these programs include special classes for parents as well. Students learn to harness emotions productively, so that classroom disruption, fighting, suspensions, and expulsions decrease, while self-control, assertiveness, problem-solving, and cooperation increase. There is a special emphasis in *Healthy People 2000* on teaching nonviolent conflict resolution skills to children in elementary and secondary schools; the goal is to increase to at least 50% the proportion of schools that teach these skills. However, it is unlikely that the goal will be achieved by 2000. Many teachers and parents are still unaware that programs to promote emotional competence exist. And our world is still populated with far too many emotionally illiterate individuals. In fact, there is a worldwide trend for the present generation of children to be more troubled emotionally than the last: more depressed, nervous, angry, and aggressive (Goleman, 1995).

I see my book as one tiny square of the quilt that is being pieced together by psychologists, teachers, social workers, nurses, and other helping professionals to address emotional health. While many of Goleman's recommendations pertain to preventive programs for children, I write for you, my colleagues, who are depressed, nervous, and angry during this turbulent time. I like to think of this quilt pulled around the shoulders of those who are crying and warming those whose emotions are cold and numb because it hurts too much to feel anymore. I hope that by the time you finish this book, your emotional reactions to events will be less distressing. I want to give you hope. It is not too late to grow and change. In contrast to old ideas that everything important is set in concrete in early childhood, we now know that emotional development continues in adulthood. Adult emotional development involves both the acquisition of new emotional habits and the abandonment, or diminished use, of old ones. Much more attention is being given by scientists and therapists to cognitive processing of emotions.

COGNITIVE PROCESSING

The term cognitive processing refers to thoughts we have before an event (our *expectations*) and thoughts after the event (our *appraisal* of what happened). Both expectations and appraisals can generate quite a lot of emotion. Let's take a situation in which a nurse named Alice is angry because she is left to pick up the pieces when others did not complete their work properly. While we can certainly view such a situation sympathetically, Alice's cognitive processing makes matters worse. For starters, her expectation is that "these idiots can't do anything right." With this expectation, she is primed for anger from the very beginning. Alice's internal dialogue runs like this: "I'll bet I am going to have to clean up their mess again. It isn't fair. I do my work; why do I have to do more than my share?" Sure enough, her prophecy is confirmed. Now appraisal comes into play. Alice makes a judgment that her coworkers are lazy or careless, thereby stoking the anger fire so that it burns ever more brightly. In this example, it's easy to see that both the expectation and the appraisal fuel excess anger. There's a lot of pejorative labeling: The other workers are thought of as incompetent "idiots," and their behavior is construed as "lazy" or "careless." Not only does Alice have to pick up the pieces today, she "always" has to do so. The other characters in the story have no redeeming features, while the nurse herself is virtuous: "I do my work." Furthermore, she rates herself favorably with regard to the quantity of work (she does more than her share) and makes an invidious comparison about the quality of the work, because the others "can't do anything right."

In contrast to earlier depictions of anger as a primitive force that may seize us, or a knee-jerk response to a stimulus, cognitive theorists say we become angry only after our brains have processed a situation sufficiently to label it an offense. For example, Novaco (1985) asserted that "there is no direct relationship between external events and anger. The arousal of anger is a cognitively mediated process" (p. 210). Within the cognitive tradition, which is relatively new, beliefs regarding the meaning of an event are crucial determinants of emotional experience. Psychologist Carol Tavris provides a delightful example:

> *One afternoon, as I was leaving the subway at rush hour, trudging tiredly up the stairs, I felt a hand brush my rear. It was an ambiguous gesture, considering the size of the crowd, so I did nothing, but my heart began to pound and my face flushed. I felt a mixture of excitement (my first New York pervert! Wait'll I tell the gang!) and fury (how dare this creep molest me). The hand struck again, this time unmistakably a pinch. I spun around, umbrella poised to strike a blow for womanhood and self-respect . . . and stared face-to-face at my husband. (Tavris, 1982, pp. 87–88)*

Our beliefs can make a situation worse because they are not always rational, which brings us to the work of Albert Ellis, founder of rational-emotive therapy (later called rational-emotive-behavior therapy). Perhaps more than any other individual, Ellis has confronted us with the irrationality of much of our thinking, and he has been doing so for more than 40 years. While I disagree with his oft-stated premise that anger is always negative and always stems from irrational beliefs, I credit him for his enormous influence on psychology and psychiatric nursing. His fundamental thesis—that thinking is a basic cause of emotion, and that healthy and unhealthy emotional reactions are significantly affected by changes in people's cognitions—has been validated by many studies (Ellis, 1973). Because of Ellis, we understand that people do not get upset but instead upset themselves. We recognized the naivete of behaviorism's stimulus-response paradigm, which wrongly concluded that external events caused people's responses. Unlike laboratory rats, humans think about and interpret stimuli and make their responses accordingly. Of course, the response of interest to us in this chapter is anger. One way of defusing anger is to challenge the irrational beliefs that trigger it.

IRRATIONAL BELIEFS AND ANGER AROUSAL

A belief is irrational if it is demanding, rigid, inaccurate, and unhelpful in assisting people to achieve their goals (Walen, DiGiuseppe, & Wessler, 1980). Let's examine some beliefs that are irrational and do not serve us well. Psychologist Melvin Lerner (1980) said that many of us have a need to believe in a Just World where the good people are rewarded and the bad people are punished. When events challenge that belief, we search for an explanation that somehow preserves it. For example, if a coworker is fired, we tell ourselves he must have deserved it. Or we might console ourselves by deciding that he will grow and become a better person through this negative experience. Our need to think there is a Just World is so great that we will blame ourselves for an event rather than relinquish the belief. For example, parents of terminally ill children may berate themselves—"If we had only done this . . ." or "We shouldn't have done that"—because it is unthinkable that a child should suffer in a Just World. But the world is *not* just. To expect it to be is ultimately an untenable expectation.

Another widely held belief, at least, in Western cultures, is that each of us has a tremendous amount of personal control over stressors, mental and physical health, social situations, and so on. Several decades of research on "internal locus of control" (a construct invented by researchers to describe belief in the personal controllability of outcomes) convinced many of us that control is quite a good thing. The literature generally portrayed "internals" as more competent, effective persons who take responsibility for their actions and take steps to change aversive situations. Training programs were established to teach people how to be "internals," as opposed to being "externals," who believed that events in their lives occurred due to fate, luck, or chance. But scientists are rethinking the concept of control these days (Shapiro, Schwartz, & Astin, 1996). There are some negative aspects of seeking and having control. Research shows that many people overestimate the amount of control they have in a situation (Seligman, 1991) and underestimate the risks associated with their behavior (Weinstein, 1984). It can be particularly detrimental to have a high desire for control in an environment that will not permit it. Anger can be fueled by futile attempts to control events that are uncontrollable.

People are notoriously uncontrollable too. Enormous energy is wasted when we try to control the behavior of our coworkers and significant others. It is irrational to believe that other people should act in accordance with our standards of behavior. When someone acts in a way that violates our belief system, we often find ourselves making judgments such as "Nobody has a right to act that way" or "He should have done such-and-such." To counter this tendency, Deffenbacher (1995b) reminds us of the "paradox of freedom": If *we* have the right to make choices (even if dumb), so too do our coworkers, friends, and family members (even if dumb and dumber). We are abridging others' freedom if we insist that everything should be done our way.

Let's not forget patients in this discussion of control. Nursing scholar Myra Levine wrote an insightful paper back in 1970 that I have held on to for all these years. Her topic: the intransigent patient, that is, the patient we cannot control, who is unwilling to follow "explicitly and faithfully, every instruction given him for 'his own good' " (1970, p. 2106). Some of the factors involved in our poor tolerance for the intransigent patient are moral indignation, personal anxiety, and guilt. There is an unrealistic premise that patients can be taught unquestioning obedience. But patients are captive students who may not want to learn what we have to teach—or do what *we* think they should do. They may not want to learn about an unappetizing low-salt, low-fat, high-fiber diet even if we think they *should* care about their heart health. Levine pleads for nurses to adopt more realistic expectations. She decries the arrogance that pervades nursing: that patients do not know what is good for them. The nurse views patients as his or hers, but patients must remain true to themselves if they are to survive. We need to drop the *shoulds* and *oughts* from our vocabulary regarding patients.

Shoulds and *oughts* are also quite frequent in our self-talk. Many of these imperatives pertain to unrealistic standards for our own performance. We believe that our self-worth is contingent on our performance. I have graduate students who castigate themselves if they do not make an A on every paper. They show up at my office to plead that a B+ or A- be changed to an A, despite my assurance that a B+ or A- grade indicates that they have done fine work. I try to point out that it is an irrational expectation that every paper should be evaluated as excellent in a rigorous nursing graduate program. But we faculty are self-critical too. As we drive home from work, reviewing our own actions, we often harshly criticize, telling ourselves, "I should have . . ." Some of us find ourselves heavily "should-on," as one humorist puts it.

An irrational belief that we identified in our study of female nurses was their notion—or fantasy—that someone should rescue them from their difficulties (Smith et al., 1996). Nurses said things like "I kind of wish the system would change" or "We don't seem to have the leadership." Some expected to be rescued by management even though they had not made their needs known. They became angry when help was not forthcoming. For example, Fran Erwin related, *"We were short-staffed, we were not getting any support, nobody really cared. . . . I had not come out and said to the supervisor, 'We need some help,' but she was aware of the census and what was going on. I blew up."* A bit later in the interview, Fran contrasted this "uncaring" supervisor who had failed to come to the rescue with her "lifesaver" who had been out of town: *"My lifesaver, resource person [the nurse manager] was not in town that week . . . she'd have found some help."*

While we can sympathize with Fran for having to work short-staffed, at no point in her narrative is there any evidence that she considered taking action herself. Fran may have been operating under another irrational assumption: that nothing could be done. What could she have done? Well, at the very least, she could have made a direct request to the supervisor for some assistance rather than assuming that the supervisor must be aware of her need. It was illogical to merely wait for someone in authority to come to the rescue. In a clever article about games nurses play, Roberts (1986) called this the "Pass to a Higher Authority" game. Players in this game speak of "they," not "I" or "we." They refer every issue to someone in a position of higher authority. Interestingly, the male nurses we studied don't seem to be involved in this game. Although there were many commonalities between female and male nurses in our studies, this irrational belief was typical only of females. Socialization to the feminine gender role inculcates the belief that if one waits patiently, a handsome prince or fairy godmother will magically appear and make things right. My friends, it's time we shelve the fairy tales.

Shelving ineffective complaining should be next on our "to do" list. Another irrational belief held by many nurses is that complaining gets results. While direct and clear anger expression is rare, complaining is rampant in nursing. Gripe sessions occupy most of our lunch and coffee breaks, and all too often pervade our after-hours socializing when we should be putting work out of our minds. Complaining actually preserves the status quo, because as long as we just complain to each other, nothing changes. Maya Angelou's grandmother taught her a valuable lesson about complaining: "What you're supposed to do when you don't like a thing is change it. If you can't change it, change the way you think about it. Don't complain" (Angelou, 1993 cited in Curtin, 1995, p. 8). Changing our thinking can defuse a lot of nonproductive anger.

All of the following are irrational beliefs held by many nurses, and I'm sure you won't have any trouble adding to this list:

1. Good nurses work until they drop—and do overtime or double shifts PRN.
2. Good nurses don't make errors.
3. Other nurses should do their work the way it "ought" to be done— that is, the way that I would do it.
4. Patients should be cooperative and grateful for our ministrations.
5. Patients should be interested in what we want to teach them about self-care.
6. Patients' families should be attentive to their loved ones but stay out of our way.

How do these irrational beliefs connect to anger? In the ABC framework of Ellis's (1973) rational emotive therapy, A is the activating event (for example, a patient complains about the nurse's care), B is the belief ("Patients should be grateful; I'm working my tail off here"), and C is the consequence ("I'm really furious at this ungrateful patient"). In this example, holding the belief that patients should be grateful is clearly a problem. Instead of exploring the patient's complaint in an empathic way, which might reveal his or her fears about helplessness or abandonment, this nurse responds angrily. What is important here is to understand that A does not cause C, because the disturbed angry feelings are primarily generated by B, the irrational belief. Research evidence (Hazaleus & Deffenbacher, 1985) supports the association between faulty thinking and anger arousal. Statistically significant correlations have been found between anger arousal and all of these irrational beliefs:

1. I must have love and approval from others.
2. I must be perfect—and consider myself worthless if a mistake is made.
3. People should be blamed and punished when they do wrong.
4. It is a catastrophe when things are not as one would like them to be.
5. Unhappiness is caused by external circumstances that are beyond one's control.
6. Possible negative events should be worried over constantly.
7. The influence of past events can never be changed or removed.
8. For every problem there is always a perfect solution that must be found.

If you groaned a bit in self-recognition as I reviewed these irrational beliefs, it's not too late to alter your mindset. Psychologist and philosopher William James observed, "The greatest revolution in our generation is the discovery that human beings, by changing their inner attitudes of their minds, can change the outer aspects of their lives." Well-known nursing author and leader Barbara Barnum has some excellent advice on altering your mindset so that you are no longer aroused to anger by irrational expectations:

> *The anger response is certainly addictive. It probably resides in some conceptualization that the world, our employers, our friends "owe" us something or some particular way of behaving. Life works better, I believe, if most of one's expectations are for oneself, not for others. Yes, I am one of*

those "we create our own worlds" people. In essence, my philosophy is to avoid an anger response, which is helped by seeing life as a school in which things are designed for character formation, not for ease of passage. I've recently recovered from an excruciating rupture of a disk, C6–C7, and I was profoundly grateful to escape surgery. The first two people I met on returning to work asked, wasn't I mad to have had such a bad injury? It's all in the mind, isn't it?

Steps Toward Healing

1. Try cognitive restructuring when your anger is generated by irrational thoughts. Begin with self-monitoring to identify biases or distortions. Write down the thoughts you have during anger episodes for a week. Look for absolute terms in your thought patterns: always, never, must, etc. Dispute these thoughts. Then develop and rehearse new cognitions that decrease the anger. A more rational cognitive appraisal can mediate the effect that an event has on your behavior. Many situations can be reinterpreted in a more positive light. At the very least, you can relabel a situation in neutral terms. As you catch yourself thinking irrationally, correct yourself (Hazaleus & Deffenbacher, 1986; Moon & Eisler, 1983; Novaco, 1975). Here are some specific tips:

   - If you tend to catastrophize ("This is the worst thing that's ever happened"), substitute more realistic thoughts such as these:

     "I'll do what I can. If it works, great. If not, well, I did the best I can."
     "Getting all bent out of shape doesn't help."
     "It's not the end of the world."

   - If you tend to demand that others behave in a certain way ("They should have done that"), substitute the following:

     "This is not what I would prefer, but I can't always expect people to act the way I want them to."
     "I don't really know why he/she did that. Maybe I need to ask."

   - If you blow things out of proportion ("I'm never going to get over this"), try to stay with a more realistic appraisal:

     "This is negative, but it's not that big a deal. No need to make myself all upset about this."
     "All things considered, this is pretty small."

- If you engage in one-track thinking ("They are doing that deliberately to get to me"), try to consider other explanations:

"Maybe they didn't know."
"I may not have all the facts."

- If you tend to apply derogatory labels ("bitch," "jerk," "idiot"),
realize that humans are too complex to be given a single global
rating. Even if behavior in a particular incident is clearly repre-
hensible and deserves condemnation, most people are not rot-
ten to the core. Try to substitute a more nuanced evaluation of
the other person:

"Maybe he's having a bad day."
*"I better not make a global judgment about him on the basis of one
incident."*

A final tip: Some people find it helpful to write rational self-
statements such as these on 3 × 5 cards for quick review until they
have been committed to memory (Dryden, 1990). You will need to
practice thinking differently in real-world situations of interpersonal conflict and criticism.

2. If you are troubled by a particular obsessive thought that you cannot banish, try thought stopping. This procedure was developed
by Cautela in 1969. The principle behind the procedure is that if
the thought is consistently interrupted whenever it occurs, its occurrence will eventually be eliminated. There are two steps:

- Close your eyes and deliberately think the unwanted thought
- As you begin to think the specific thought, shout "Stop!" Do
this 10 or 20 times a day for 2 or 3 days. Then move to a modifi-
cation of the procedure where you say "Stop" to yourself, rather
than aloud, every other time you practice. Then say "Stop" to
yourself every single time. After a few days of practice, you
should be able to halt the unwanted thought whenever it begins.

3. Make a greater effort to understand the other person's point of
view or motives. In a very interesting study, participants in a conflict were asked to provide narratives about their anger experience. Angry people nearly always insisted that the other person's
behavior was wrong, while their own was justified. They described
the offenders' actions as unreasonable, arbitrary, selfish, even malicious. The offenders did not see their actions in this way at all

and offered coherent and reasonable explanations of their motivation and behavior. Descriptions of the incidents were entirely different. The individuals who had been angered described the incidents in long-term contexts, with few extenuating circumstances and lasting adverse consequences. The offenders held a much more benign view of things. While acknowledging that they had done wrong, the offenders minimized the severity of the incidents. In their view, the angry incidents were time-limited, with mitigating circumstances and happy endings. The researchers concluded that anger is characterized by "a gap in interpersonal understanding" (Baumeister, Stillwell, & Wotman, 1990). I would say that's putting it mildly!

I am reminded of a conflict between two students who were working together on a project. One of them had come to me on several occasions to express her resentment at the perceived lack of interest on the part of the other student. In her view, the other student had little intrinsic investment in the project and was contributing in a minimal, perfunctory manner. In due time, the "accused" showed up to tell me her side of the story. The words rapidly tumbled out as she recounted her extreme frustration, especially with the "do-it-at-the-last-minute" style of the other student. I soon gained an appreciation of the conflict from her perspective, which was quite different from the impression I had initially formed. Each student made some very valid points. There was no clear "right" or "wrong," just two very different personalities and styles of getting work done.

I have learned that behavior that ticks me off can often be explained, at least in part, by differences in tempo (turtles vs. racehorses), need for order in the environment (neatniks vs. slobs), or ways of thinking (left brain vs. right brain). I give my students the Myers-Briggs Type Inventory so they will have a better understanding of personality. There is much potential for conflict within a work group because different personality types are bewildered by one another. For example, introverts can't imagine why extraverts have to talk all the time. Extraverts can't fathom why introverts need time alone to recharge their batteries. Logical analysts are puzzled by the deeply emotional, and so forth. With a better understanding of personality, we are more likely to appreciate and value our opposites.

Finally, I have learned a tremendous amount from two of my friends. Because I am very logical and goal-directed, I plunge ahead with my eye on the goal, taking the most efficient way to get there. I am not looking at the flowers as I go, much less taking time to smell them. Time is important to me: being on time and using time wisely. My friends are almost always late to our meetings, blissfully unaware of time passing. They are looking at the scenery, chatting with passersby, and appreciating things that I miss completely in my rush to get to my destination. Rather than getting angry at their lateness, I have learned from their relaxed orientation toward time and their esthetic sensitivities, and they have learned to tolerate my impatience to move on. Sometimes, it is an uneasy truce, because we are very different, but our friendship is important. What helps is that we are able to talk freely with one another. If you work with someone who infuriates you, consider what his or her view of your conflict might be. It is unlikely that this person is deliberately trying to make your life miserable. Wouldn't it be interesting to explore his or her interpretation of the conflict? Give it a try.

When you have relinquished the "I'm right-and-they're-wrong" view of anger incidents, it's time for another step in the journey toward improved emotional health. Read on.

4

Modifying Nonproductive Anger Styles

What do nurses do when they are angered on the job?

> *"I stood there and took it. It's kind of like kicking a dog and the dog never runs off."*
> *"I was screaming at my nurse manager. I got frustrated and angry and screamed at her."*
> *"I go to the medicine room and cuss."*
> *"I kind of back off."*
> *"I really blow up and I start crying. I feel better it's out, but I wish I had handled it a little better."*

None of these nurses felt good about how they handled their anger. In fact, most nurses I've talked to about work-related anger incidents echo that last statement: They wish they had handled their anger a little better. Learning to modify a nonproductive anger style can be one of the most important self-management projects you will ever undertake. Both your career and your health will benefit, and the profession itself will benefit. Some nurses are harboring their anger until, like a malignant growth, it chokes the love of nursing out of them. Feeling powerless to effect change and giving up the hope of being rescued, they leave—either physically, by changing employers or professions, or mentally, by remaining on the job but merely going through the motions. They are the dispirited walking wounded in every health care setting. Beverly Malone, president of the American Nurses Association, had this to say:

Nurses have a legitimate right to be angry, but along with that right come consequences and challenges. The goal is not to eliminate anger but to acknowledge it and channel it into positive, life-supporting interventions. Acknowledging the anger will remind nurses of how far they have to go; programmatically channeling the anger will remind nurses of how far they have already come. (Malone, 1985, p. 45)

Why change your anger behavior? Because if you continue to do what you've always done, you'll get what you've always gotten. You must have some dissatisfaction with the status quo, or you wouldn't be reading this book. I like Bev Malone's emphasis on "positive, life-supporting interventions." That is my emphasis throughout this book. Anger *can* be controlled and channeled into constructive actions that improve your work life and your relationships. But most people simply don't know how. The research of Dianne Tice (1990) is informative. In a free-format response questionnaire, more than 400 men and women were asked about their strategies for controlling, and altering, negative emotional states such as sadness, fear, anxiety, and anger. For each emotional state, the study participants were asked if they had tried to change it while experiencing it, and if so, how. People had fewer strategies for controlling anger than for the other emotions, and they viewed their strategies as less successful than the strategies they used to control other emotions. Tice's findings should not surprise us, given the difficulties we see in our society with anger management. There is a pervasive notion in American culture that anger is involuntary, that it is not controllable.

How did we get such an idea? It is derived from influences of Darwinian evolutionary theory, Freudian theory, and research on aggression in animals. In this view, anger is considered a powerful instinctive drive. Therefore, holding it back or bottling it up is deemed unhealthy because it will eventually erupt in some form. According to Weiner (1991), the metaphor of machine is applicable to this view. A machine has a fixed amount of energy; if energy is spent performing one function, it will be unavailable for others. The language of hydraulics is evident in Freud's terms *cathexis* (filling) and *catharsis* (release). Although Freud himself never recommended the full-blown overt expression of anger for catharsis, others within the psychodynamic tradition have done so. Irate individuals are urged to "get in touch with those feelings," or "let it all hang out." So-called catharsis is allegedly achieved by ventilation. In the 1970s, a number of people became involved in encounter groups and other therapies that encouraged expression of their pent-up feelings. I remember patients on psychiatric units being told by staff to pound pillows, rip up telephone books, and throw bean bags to "get the anger out." In a 1974 book called *Creative Aggression*, readers were actually advised to insult, scold, and scream at other people. The authors also recommended the formation of "insult clubs" and "family aggression festivals" (Bach & Goldberg, 1974). During this period of time, primal scream therapy was the latest rage—literally!

But there was virtually no empirical testing of the efficacy of these ways of managing anger. In fact, until the era of behavioral and cognitive-behavioral therapies, there was a dearth of research on anger interventions of any kind. Research in the 1980s and 1990s has not supported the idea that ventilation is an unequivocal good. Psychotherapy clients who demonstrate the most catharsis don't necessarily demonstrate the greatest change (Safran & Greenberg, 1991). As Gendlin (1973) pointed out, "If you are living in an intolerable situation, no amount of catharting will exhaust your anger; it will arise anew every time you are in, or put yourself into, the situation" (p. 385). Explosive venting of anger actually makes a person angrier rather than having a cathartic effect. Try this experiment the next time you're furious: Yell at the top of your lungs and note your physiological arousal. Keep yelling. Are you getting the anger off your chest or fueling more of it? I think you'll find that anger fuels more anger. You can also conduct this experiment when someone is yelling at you. Yell back. Turn the volume up. Chances are, the other person will also turn up the volume. Infuriating, isn't it? As the conflict escalates, are you feeling better or worse?

It is a cultural myth that you'll feel better if you respond to other people's anger with a vociferous blast—"giving back as good as you got," as the saying goes. There is an interesting study of men and women who give traffic tickets in New York City. You can imagine how unpopular these workers are, and how often they are bombarded by angry motorists who just got a ticket. The study showed that the workers who responded angrily to confrontation were more upset afterward. In contrast, those who used a calm conflict management style felt better about the way they handled the confrontation (Brondolo, Bendetto, Storrs, Baruch, & Contrada, 1993).

There is a new view that stands in stark contrast to the shout-it-out ventilationist school of thought: I call this one the stuff-it-in stoic approach. This approach has gained prominence because of the compelling research on the overtly angry coronary-prone personality over the past two decades. It is clear that unrestrained ventilation could be dangerous, even fatal. Thus, anger has been labeled by some as a toxic emotion. One recent book was given the sensational title *Anger Kills*

(Williams & Williams, 1993). Its authors claim that getting angry is like "taking a small dose of some slow-acting poison—arsenic, for example" (p. xiii), and they recommend that anger be "cut off" (p. xvi). And so the pendulum has swung to the other extreme: This lethal poison must be controlled.

The stuff-it-in stoic view is not really new. The Stoic philosophers thought emotions caused misery and therefore must be harnessed. Typical of their advice are these words from Seneca (a Roman philosopher born in 4 B.C.): "Hesitation is the best cure for anger." Similarly, an old Chinese proverb advocates patience: "If you are patient in one moment of anger, you will escape a hundred days of sorrow" (cited in Seldes, 1985). Once again, hesitation and patience are in vogue. Not only are the old maxims like "Count to 10" being revived, but the new line of advice to the public is "Just don't get angry." In my opinion, this simplistic advice is about as useful as Nancy Reagan's slogan "Just say no to drugs." In the Women's Anger Study (Thomas, 1993b), anger occurred mainly in dyadic encounters with intimates (spouses, children, friends, or coworkers) who had behaved disrespectfully or irresponsibly. It seems unrealistic that anger within these close interpersonal relationships could ever be eradicated. And suppressing it practically guarantees that it will take a devious course, ultimately causing relationship damage because the anger-provoking issue has never been worked through. As I emphasize throughout this book, anger has useful functions in self-protection and correction of injustices.

There is another experiment that I recommend to you. The next time something makes you angry, try to abort the emotion. Stuff it, squelch it, try to make it go away. What happens? I think you will find that when you suppress it, is the physiological arousal is prolonged, along with rumination about the grievance that provoked the anger. So it doesn't go away. There is a nagging unrest because you have not acted on your true feelings. And suppression of anger, as we have seen in Chapter 2, is linked to higher blood pressure and a number of other physical health problems. Avoidance of painful emotion is considered the core of many mental health problems as well (Perls, Hefferline, & Goodman, 1951). As Peter Whybrow (1997) puts it: *"Emotion is an instrument of self correction—when we are happy or sad, it has meaning. Seeking ways to blot out variation in mood is equivalent to an airline pilot ignoring his navigational devices"* (p. 72).

Reviewing the conflicting advice that abounds in the literature, many of us are left wondering what we are supposed to *do* with our anger. Neither shouting it out nor stuffing it in contributes to improved relationships with coworkers or family members, and neither is good for our own health. Nor should we turn anger on ourselves, making self-deprecating comments like "What a fool I was for trusting her" or "I'm furious with myself for accepting that assignment in the first place." Isn't there a rational alternative? That is what we are going to talk about now.

ANGER DISCUSSION

There *is* a way to handle anger that is adaptive and health-promoting, although it has received much less scrutiny by scientists. Consistent with everything else in medical and behavioral science, the focus has been on pathology rather than health. Thus, researchers have mainly studied the two extreme modes of expression you've just read about: "anger-in" and "anger-out." The earliest mention in the research literature of a healthier way of expressing anger is in 1979, in a study by Harburg, Blakelock, and Roeper. The researchers described a reflective anger coping style that was used to handle an angry boss. The style involved inhibiting impulsive reactions, waiting until the heat of the anger had cooled, then having a rational discussion. Individuals who used this method had lower blood pressures compared with those who held anger inside or expressed anger outwardly. Interestingly, females were more likely to choose this approach than males were.

About the same time as the Harburg paper, the first reports of the Framingham Heart Study were surfacing (Haynes, Feinleib, Levine, Scotch, & Kannel, 1978; Haynes, Levine, Scotch, Feinleib, & Kannel, 1978). Along with "anger-in" and "anger-out," the investigative team had measured a rational alternative: "anger-discuss," which involved getting anger off one's chest through discussion of the incident with a friend or relative. Subsequently, I have chosen the Framingham Anger Scales for a number of my own studies because I wanted my study participants to have the opportunity to say whether they used this adaptive anger management style as well as holding their anger in or venting it outwardly. Coming from a nursing perspective, I wanted to know what behavior would be health promoting rather than focusing exclusively on what is health damaging.

Through the years I have found that the only anger expression style correlated positively to general physical health is anger-discuss (Thomas & Williams, 1991). Anger discussion is also correlated positively with self-esteem (Saylor & Denham, 1993), and it is inversely correlated with stress (Thomas & Donnellan, 1993) and depression (Droppleman &

Wilt, 1993). In other words, you feel better about yourself and experience less stress and depression when you get anger off your chest. Other research findings are encouraging too. One of my doctoral students found that anger discussion is correlated with a stronger sense of self-efficacy and optimism (Ausbrooks, Thomas, & Williams, 1995). In my most recent piece of research, involving over 400 men and women, ages 18 to 77, I compared anger discussers (those who say they usually discuss their anger) with nondiscussers (those who do not usually discuss anger). Discussers had lower systolic and diastolic blood pressures and lower body mass index (an obesity indicator). Additionally, discussers were more likely than nondiscussers to value their health highly, perceive better current health status, and engage in regular aerobic exercise (Thomas, 1997a). Findings of these studies are consistent with research by James Pennebaker (1992) on the beneficial health effects of sharing feelings about troubling events. Whether disclosed to a human listener or to a tape recorder, the verbalization of emotion resulted in better immune system function and fewer visits to health care providers.

When the anger-discuss mode is included in the tests researchers administer, women consistently score higher than men (Riley, Treiber, & Woods, 1989; Thomas, 1989, 1997a; Thomas & Williams, 1991; Weidner, Istvan, & McKnight, 1989). Similarly, James Averill (1982) found that women, more so than men, wanted to talk about angry incidents, either with the instigator or with a third party. The greater propensity of females to discuss their anger with another person has been documented as early as fourth grade. In a study of boys and girls from 4th, 8th, and 12th grades, Brondolo (1992) found that girls at all ages were more willing than boys to confide in someone about their angry feelings. In summary, this gender difference has been confirmed in hundreds of adults from ages 18 to 77 and in at least one study of children and adolescents. Discussion of anger is more difficult for men because of their gender role socialization. Miller (1983) contended that fathers have not built a base of exchange of emotions with their sons. Instead of talking, boys have been encouraged to discharge anger in motor action such as fistfights. As adults, males continue to display more physical aggression than females (Deffenbacher, 1994). Later, we will talk more about gender differences (see Chapter 7), but for now, let me bring you up to date on recent developments in the research on adaptive anger.

In addition to the "Anger-discuss" scale, researchers have some new tools to measure adaptive anger. Charlie Spielberger (1988) introduced a scale measuring "anger control" that includes tendencies to be patient and calm when angry, lessening one's cognitive and emotional arousal. A "Reciprocal Communication" scale has been developed by

Jerry Deffenbacher (1994) to assess expressing one's thoughts and opinions clearly and tactfully, asking others for their opinions (and listening to them), and working toward compromise solutions. Studies using the new scales show that when people use these rational modes of anger management, they are less likely to suffer a variety of adverse consequences. Anger control and reciprocal communication are negatively correlated with depression and anxiety, alcohol use, property damage, and damaged friendships (Deffenbacher, Oetting, Lynch, & Morris, 1996).

If we apply the findings of these studies, we can learn how to behave more effectively when provoked to anger. The work situation may be bad, but we will be in a better position to cope with it. Simply put, what the research suggests to the angry individual is talking, in a normal tone, about the grievance. Ideally, direct discussion takes place with the other person. I do realize that this is not always possible due to situational constraints. When we are at work, we often need to remain calm and pleasant to patients and persons in authority, even if we are boiling inside. We are not unlike flight attendants in this regard, a group that must suppress their anger at demanding and obnoxious passengers. Hochschild (1979) studied this group, finding that the flight attendants experienced considerable emotional problems. Some reported that they felt emotionally "numb" because of the continual suppression of annoyance, irritation, and anger. The researcher speculated that any individual in an occupation with strong rules inhibiting anger will experience difficulties similar to flight attendants.

But as we can see from the burgeoning research literature, we cannot afford to remain silent in our emotional discomfort. When discussion cannot take place with the provocateur, we need to find a confidant such as a good friend and unburden ourselves. This gets the anger out harmlessly. There are a number of other benefits. Discussion is:

- a healthy way to review what happened
- an effective method for obtaining empathy and feedback
- a good means of formulating ideas to solve problems

However, there is a caution. As you talk about the incident with your confidant, you do not want to prolong or escalate your anger. So avoid raising your voice, pounding your fist, and using profanity. And choose someone who will listen attentively but not fuel additional anger by making inflammatory comments. As I mentioned in an earlier chapter, it is not helpful if the other person injects his or her own views. Select someone who was not involved in the anger-producing episode and has no built-in bias or prejudice about any aspect of it. For example, if your anger is directed at a doctor, you would not want to tell your story to a person who is known to hate doctors. Your goal is to get the anger off your chest and let it go.

While getting anger off your chest can be very therapeutic, you may be wondering how this approach can lead to resolution of the original issue. You're right, it can't.

The poet William Blake sums it up far better than I:

> I was angry with my friend:
> I told my wrath, my wrath did end.
> I was angry with my foe:
> I told it not, my wrath did grow."
>
> (cited in Seldes, *The Great Thoughts*, 1985, p. 44)

At some point you will have to take your anger to the provocateur for a one-to-one discussion that can lead to resolution of the problem. For example, if you have been treated unfairly by a supervisor, you must first cool down and reflect, then discuss your feelings about the unfair treatment with the supervisor. Your goal is to express your anger clearly and tactfully to the other person in a nonblaming way. Listen to the response and move into a bargaining mode, prepared to negotiate and compromise. Few problems are entirely one-sided.

If you are sitting here reading all of this and saying to yourself, "There's not a snowball's chance in Hades that I would be able to go to my supervisor and do that," keep on reading, because now we turn to very specific techniques to change your anger behavior. I can assure you that I have seen amazing transformations in people's emotional habits. It's never too late to undertake a behavior change project, to choose to learn and grow. I strongly believe that all of us are moving forward toward wholeness throughout life, and being able to master a wide repertoire of emotional behaviors is an important aspect of being whole persons. The first step in changing anger behavior is spelled out by one of nursing's greatest scholars, teachers, and leaders, Hildegard Peplau:

> *It is important to gain an understanding of what occurred in situations in which anger is evoked. This requires a review and analysis of interaction data, including one's own participation in the event. Control of anger, as a response in situations, flows from recognizing the anger and understanding what evoked it.*

Self-Assessment

1. As Peplau recommends, I ask you to engage in some careful introspection. I realize that focusing on oneself takes courage. It's more comfortable to find the other person at fault. But research shows that this step is a crucial one in any self-change endeavor (Williams, Pettibone, & Thomas, 1991). Anger is a confusing emotion for most of us. In the heat of an argument, we often lose track of the original provocation. Later on, with a cooler head, reflection produces some insight. I recommend keeping an anger diary or log for a month or so, recording accounts of conflictual interactions at work. If you really hate writing, an alternative way of keeping a diary of your anger episodes is tape-recording. Whether you write or make audiotapes, try to include all pertinent details about the interaction. What I am asking you to do is somewhat like the process recordings that you did as a student in psychiatric nursing or field notes that you took during a research project. Just as a researcher does, you are going to analyze the data after collecting it:

   Who provokes your anger at work? What situations or circumstances usually set you off? Do you understand why? What thoughts are going through your mind? Do other people usually know when you are angry or do you keep it inside? What themes or patterns can you find in your anger diary entries? For example, do situations of powerlessness or injustice occur over and over? Are there issues of unmet expectations or betrayal of trust? Does criticism infuriate you? Do you become angered because of events that are outside of your control? Are your diary entries peppered with "shoulds"? If you are getting angry at yourself, what messages are you giving yourself? Are there differences in the frequency or intensity of your anger lately? How long does a typical day-to-day anger episode usually last for you?

   As you review your log or diary, pay particular attention to the recurrent anger themes and patterns. And watch for signs that your anger is out of control. It is cause for concern if the anger is too frequent, too intense, or out of proportion to the transgression. It is cause for major concern if your anger has become chronic or spills over to your patients. Look carefully at the aftereffects of episodes. Are you ruminating for a long time, unable to let go of your angry thoughts and feelings?

2. Next, assess your anger expression style. While none of us behaves exactly the same way in all situations, there is usually some consis-

tency in our behavior. If your style is mainly discussing your anger in an effective, rational way, you may not need to read the rest of this chapter. What I focus on in this section are nonproductive anger expression styles. In my work, I have found that two nonproductive styles predominate. They are pretty consistent with the shout-it-out ventilationist and stuff-it-in stoic approaches that I have been talking about. These styles are termed by researchers "anger-out" and "anger-in." But when I am making presentations to the public, I usually refer to the "garlic people" and the "onion people." I'm not sure where I first heard about this typology, but I have used it in workshops ever since. The "onion people" swallow most of their anger, and just as individuals who eat onions suffer inner distress afterward, so do these anger suppressors. There's an aftertaste, and the anger just keeps trying to come back up. In contrast, the "garlic people," who freely spread overt anger all around, cause others to suffer, often for a prolonged time. But the garlic eater is no longer aware of the smell. He or she is just fine. Which are you?

You are an anger suppressor—an "onion person"—if several of the following statements describe your behavior, at least on some occasions:

> I become anxious when my anger is aroused.
> When angry, I try to act as though nothing happened.
> I keep my anger to myself.
> I boil inside, but do not show it.
> I am angrier than I am willing to admit.
> I ruminate, pout, or sulk.
> I harbor grudges.
> I withdraw from people.
> I convey anger through an icy stare, frown, or "a look that could kill."
> I convey anger by rolling my eyes or raising my eyebrows.
> I convey anger through body language (folding arms, putting hands on hips, etc.).
> I convey anger through the "silent treatment"

You are a "garlic person" if several of the following statements describe your behavior, at least on some occasions:

> I become argumentative.
> I fly off the handle.

I throw things.
I strike out at whatever infuriates me.
I slam doors.
I raise my voice, scream or yell.
I tell people off.
I say nasty things.
I lose my temper.
I hit or break things.
I call the other person names.
I stomp around.

Steps Toward Healing for Those Who Direct Anger Inward

1. If you assessed yourself to be an "onion person," you may be so accustomed to denying or disavowing your anger that you are not even sure when you're angry. You may need to become more closely attuned to your bodily signals of distress or the defense mechanisms that automatically shunt your anger elsewhere as soon as it's generated. Defenses such as repression, denial, projection, isolation, or intellectualization may have served you well for a long time. It may take a while to give them up. You may have learned that anger is a sin, a notion that I disputed in Chapter 3. Some anger suppressors do not like the word *anger*, preferring to minimize their emotional arousal by using weaker terms. For example, they may say they are "a little irritated" or "kinda upset." Does this ring true for you? If so, your first assignment is to "own" the emotion of anger and add the word *anger* to your vocabulary. Recognizing, naming, and honoring your legitimate anger is important. Set incremental goals for yourself. For example, begin by changing your self-talk: "It's all right to be angry." Then work on saying—out loud—"I am angry" instead of "I'm kinda upset."

2. Learn to experience and express anger. Give yourself permission to do so. You are not truly free until you are unafraid to feel each emotion, including anger. When anger is inhibited, it just rolls up into a big ball, as one of our study participants described: "It's like you build up so much anger inside . . . without really sitting down and talking about the problem . . . it just rolls up into a big ball and you're not even sure what it's really about." This woman's metaphor conjures up an image of a multicolored ball of yarn, a tangled skein of grievances that have accumulated for a long time. If you've been rolling all your anger and aggravation into a big

ball like this, it may be frightening to contemplate unraveling it. Be assured that you don't have to do it all at once. Nor am I urging you to begin using anger to confront all of your problems. I have seen women go from marshmallow to Medusa after a few sessions of assertiveness training. That's *not* what we're about. What you *will* need to learn is to express anger at the time of its provocation rather than hiding it, ruminating about the grievance, and connecting it to a host of past grievances, so that another big ball of anger begins to accumulate. In the words of George Schrader (1973): "Anger is better disposed of as it arises in the commonplace situations of everyday life. What we need is to be free *for* our anger rather than to be free *from* it" (p. 349).

3. Realize that anger is not catastrophic. Women who participated in our phenomenological study of anger (Thomas et al., in press) feared they would alienate others if they expressed their feelings. Anger was viewed as something that "breaks the circle" of the relationship, as one woman phrased it. Another study participant said, "I guess I'm afraid that if I express anger I will be rejected because I'm expressing myself and my needs, and I feel like if I do express needs at all . . . I'll be rejected." In our studies of nurses, males as well as females reported withdrawal from coworkers for fear of catastrophic consequences (Brooks et al., 1996; Smith et al., 1996). However, research by James Averill (1983) showed that relationships are strengthened, not weakened, by an honest expression of anger. Targets of anger often gained rather than lost respect for the angry person. I like the metaphor of a short circuit to describe an angry encounter between persons. Wires pop and sparks fly, but the connection can be restored (Schrader, 1973). In contrast, withdrawal when you are angry severs the connection and leaves the other person in the dark about what ticked you off.

4. Work through guilt about being angry. Harriet Lerner (1985) sagely notes: "Anger and guilt are just about incompatible. . . Nothing, but nothing, will block the awareness of anger so effectively as guilt. . . Nor is it easy to gain the courage to stop feeling guilty and begin to use our anger to question and define what is right and appropriate for our own lives" (pp. 6–7). Research shows that women experience more guilt about anger than men do, and our guilt has been attributed to empathy for the victim (Campbell, 1993). How do we get rid of this guilt? By expressing anger in the right way at the right time, assertively. Assertive anger expression does not hurt the other person. There is no need for guilt when anger is being

used to call attention to issues that are vitally important to us because of our values, beliefs, and rights as human beings.

5. Learn to tolerate the inhibiting responses of others when you try
out new assertive behaviors. If you have been Doris (or Don)
Doormat, your colleagues may want you to stay the same. Why
wouldn't they? They could always count on you to work a double
shift or take an extra patient. Likewise, your family didn't mind a
bit that you were the one loading the dishwasher at midnight or
going around picking up all the dirty towels on the bathroom
floor. When you start requesting them to shoulder more of the
workload, their response is predictably unenthusiastic: "What's
gotten into you?" Lerner (1985) called it the "Change back!" reaction. You may be accused of coldness or selfishness, and of course
the old guilt-button will probably get pushed.

Don't be discouraged if you meet resistance. Expect it. Remind
yourself that what you are doing is good for you, and ultimately
good for the other people who have used you as a doormat. Suppressing or turning anger inward does not prevent negative consequences. Research by Jerry Deffenbacher and his colleagues
(1996) showed that Anger-In was significantly correlated with a variety of negative consequences, including damaged friendships
and feeling physically ill and depressed. Moreover, holding anger
in was highly correlated with feeling ashamed, dumb, embarrassed,
and bad about oneself. Many of our study participants who suppressed their anger eventually erupted in volcanic outbursts that
also left them ashamed and embarrassed (Thomas et al., in press).
Here is an example from our data. A woman had simmered and
stewed about her 16-year-old son wrecking the car but said nothing. Several nights later, she was roaming the house, sleepless, ruminating about the accident—and becoming angrier at her son. At
2:00 a.m. she awakened him and blasted him: *"It was like a volcano;
once it erupts it all came out, little by little by little. I thought, 'I have just
lost control; I'm a crazy woman."* Clearly, suppressing the anger had
only postponed the inevitable confrontation with her son, and her
outburst was much more ineffective than a forthright discussion at
the time of the accident would have been. You can imagine what a
fearful sight she was to her sleepy teenager!

6. If you tend to pout, sulk, or ruminate about angry interactions for
a prolonged period, try mental flossing. As you floss your teeth at
night, you remove the food particles that will be a breeding
ground for bacteria in your mouth. In the same way that flossing

teeth leaves your mouth cleaner and less prone to gum infection or caries, mental flossing gets rid of troublesome thoughts that can "infect" your mental health. It does no good to keep thinking about what happened over and over again. Cleanse your mind and heart at bedtime.

7. If you tend to express a lot of anger through somatic symptoms (headaches, gastric distress), you need to learn to use words instead. Play detective for a few weeks, tracking the connections between getting angry at particular people or situations and the onset of these physical symptoms. How much time elapses between the feelings of irritation, tension, or fury and the headache or churning stomach? What strategy could you adopt to discharge the anger more constructively? With whom could you talk honestly about how you feel? There are many reasons why you may have difficulty in finding words for your feelings, such as early life experiences with your mother or growing up in a family that restricted emotional expression. In addition to the self-help strategies in this book, you may need the assistance of a counselor. Verbalization can be practiced in individual counseling or group therapy. You can learn to use body scanning (see Chapter 2) to identify early cues, like tense neck muscles, that anger is escalating. If you are extremely anxious about verbalizing anger, gaining control of your anxiety will be crucial. Ferreting out the source of the anxiety will probably lead back to your relationship with your parents. During the course of development, anger is felt most consistently toward parents. If they recoiled or responded harshly to your childish anger outbursts, it is understandable that anxiety accompanies anger arousal in later life. Techniques such as deep breathing and progressive muscle relaxation (see the next section for details) may be helpful in managing the anxiety that seems to go hand-in-hand with anger.

Steps Toward Healing for Those Who Direct Anger Outward

1. If you assessed yourself to be a "garlic person," your first assignment is to become less reactive. Chances are that you are getting bent out of shape too frequently and/or too intensely. You have a short fuse, and your goal will be to achieve a longer fuse and a more moderate response style. Many daily provocations are relatively trivial and should simply be ignored. They are not worth get-

ting angry about. If you cannot ignore what is happening, distract yourself. Imagery can be useful to shift your mental focus. For example, visualize an idyllic scene in the mountains, high above the petty irritations that plague you so. From this lofty vantage point, you can see the molehills for what they really are.

2. Another tactic to dispel excess anger is to find a bit of humor in a frustrating situation. Humor creates a subjective state that is incompatible with anger. Some folks already know this: Participants in Dianne Tice's (1990) study said they were more likely to use humor to control anger than to control other negative moods such as sadness. I have learned how to do this from my husband. He is good at discovering something to laugh at when circumstances are maddening. For example, when trapped in a colossal tie-up on the interstate, he began to watch the other motorists. He would call my attention to their faces, which portrayed the gamut of furious reactions to the traffic jam. People were screwing their faces into the most hideous expressions, snarling and spitting angry words into their cellular telephones. It became quite comical. We laughed, time passed, and we moved on when the accident was cleared away. It was a good lesson to me.

3. Learn calming techniques. You must reduce your physiological arousal before you can think clearly and take appropriate action on anger provocations. An excellent, simple procedure called the relaxation response was developed by Herbert Benson, a professor at Harvard Medical School. Benson (1993) asserts that many studies have shown that anger and hostility decrease in people who regularly elicit the relaxation response. Here are his instructions:

- First, make arrangements so that you will not be interrupted.
- Pick a focus word or short phrase consistent with your belief system, for example *Shalom*, or the opening words of Psalm 23.
- Sit quietly in a comfortable position.
- Close your eyes.
- Relax your muscles.
- Breathe slowly and naturally, repeating your focus word as you exhale.
- If other thoughts come to mind, gently return to the repetition of the focus word.
- Continue for 10 to 20 minutes. You may open your eyes to check the time, but do not use an alarm. When you finish, sit quietly for a minute or so. Do not stand for 1 to 2 minutes.

Another good way of cooling down is progressive muscle relaxation (PMR). Familiar to most nurses, this technique involves first tensing and then relaxing the muscles, most often from head to toe. You will need to sit in a comfortable chair or lie on a carpeted floor. Loosen tight clothing. If the technique is new to you, I recommend the purchase of an audiotape to guide you through the steps for the first few times. When you are finished with the procedure, you should feel deep calm and peace.

Still another approach is taking a time-out from the situation in which your anger is building. Taking a time-out does not mean stalking off in a huff. It means making a choice to postpone a confrontation until you can present your concerns more effectively. If possible, leave for one hour. Do not get in your automobile. We do not need any more angry drivers on the road. Instead, engage in something physical, like walking briskly. Do not return to the situation until you feel more solidly in control.

4. Assess what the real source of your anger is. There is a reason for your overreaction, although it may not be immediately evident. Your anger diary or some dream work can be helpful here. You may be surprised at what you discover. Author Gail Godwin (1983) describes her "angry year" in which she "seethed from morning till night with a hot, unspecific anger" (p. 241). Everybody infuriated her, but she did understand why. At last she identified "the Culprit." She was really angry at herself. She relates that the Culprit's "favorite trick is posing as other people whom I hate until I realize I'm hating myself" (p. 258).

5. Plan ahead to avoid negative outcomes of angry behavior. In the psychotherapy literature this is called "thinking-ahead training." First, identify the negative outcomes of your anger in a contingency statement: "If I lose my temper, I will have an upset stomach." Then, when you walk into the workplace and run smack into the very individual who drives you up the wall, remind yourself of the negative consequences and substitute alternative behavior (Feindler & Ecton, 1986).

6. Decrease ventilation. Although spouting off may be satisfying temporarily, providing you with some release of tension, it decreases your personal and professional effectiveness. When you ventilate frequently, other people are likely to say, "Oh, there she goes again!" People begin to tune you out or avoid being around you. Decide whether an issue is really important enough to respond to, then respond in a less extreme way.

7. Be assertive, not aggressive. If you prize your aggressiveness and fear that you will become a pushover or wimp without it, try reframing the aggression as weak and cowardly, while being able to stay cool and calm in negotiations is strong and powerful (Deffenbacher, 1992). You are probably accustomed to some benefits of aggressive behavior, such as getting others to comply with your demands, but keep in mind that these benefits are ultimately offset by damage to interpersonal relationships. Other people are left feeling coerced and resentful. Deffenbacher (1995b) suggests thinking about how you would want your coworkers to describe you at your retirement party. I believe that you can get much of what you want with assertiveness, with a lot less fallout. See Chapter 10 for specifics about assertive behavior.

8. Consider systematic desensitization treatment. Developed by Wolpe in 1958, this treatment involves collaborative development by the counselor and the client of a hierarchy of anger-arousing situations. Listed in the hierarchy are typical scenarios in which you experience strong reactions, ranging from the least anger-provoking to the most anger-provoking. After you learn a relaxation technique, such as progressive muscle relaxation, you use imagery to generate the anger you would customarily feel in the first scenario on the hierarchy. Then, while aroused to anger, you counteract it with relaxation. Once you have mastered anger control in the first scenario, you move on to others of progressive difficulty in the hierarchy. Systematic desensitization treatment has been shown to be highly effective in a number of studies, including two conducted with female nursing students (Evans, Hearn, & Saklofske, 1973; Hearn & Evans, 1972).

Steps Toward Healing for Everyone

Some anger management principles apply to everyone, regardless of your expression style.

I'm aware that some of you alternate between shouting it and stuffing it. The "onion" and "garlic" types are, of course, extremes of the anger continuum. So read on for other steps toward healing that are useful.

1. Take constructive action on the precipitants of your anger whenever you can. My ABCs of effective action are: *A*ssertiveness, *B*argaining, and *C*oalition-Forming (Thomas & Droppleman, 1997). Translate your anger into an assertive request (clearly stated as "I

need _____"). Bargain for better conditions. Get other nurses to join with you in a coalition to tackle a common problem. We will have more to say about taking action in Part Four.

2. If constructive action is not possible, find a private spot where you will not be interrupted—the bathroom if all else fails. Then do this short anger-releasing exercise: close your eyes, breathe deeply, and focus your attention on repeating the word "peace." Exhale your anger. Let it out. Barbara Dossey (1995) suggests the establishment of a healing room in your work site, a place for staff to go for 10 to 20 minutes to nourish themselves. In the room are comfortable pillows on a carpeted floor, beautiful pictures, and a library of music, relaxation, and imagery tapes. Such a space can also be created in your home.

3. If you tend to cry when angry, do not be ashamed or apologetic about your tears. And do not leave the interaction. Crying simply indicates that you have strong feelings, and you can say this to the other person: "I'm crying because I feel so strongly about this issue." Tears on the job are not at all unusual. Plas and Hoover-Dempsey (1988) found that 80% of women and 50% of men have cried at least once during their working lives. Although some episodes of crying resulted from sadness, the tears were an expression of anger for many people. Women cry out of anger more frequently than men, their tears emerging from the frustration that what they are saying is not being heard—or is being rejected out of hand. Ultimately, the solution to this frustration is to master the techniques in this book that will allow you to deliver verbal messages with more confidence and oomph. Hang in there because there's lots more to cover.

4. Don't displace work-related anger on the folks at home. Both "garlic" and "onion" types do this, sometimes unknowingly. The garlic person may be slamming pots and pans or snapping at the kids, while the onion person's anger may be disguised in unresponsiveness or inertia: "I'm just too tired. You go to the movies without me." Family members may be hurt and bewildered by such behavior. I recommend a decompression time during the drive home from work, to mentally "finish" with the emotional upheaval of the workday and prepare to greet your family in better spirits. Even if a work situation is infuriating or you have been treated unjustly, perpetuating an angry mood serves no good purpose. Displacing your anger onto the wrong targets cannot produce satisfaction. "Lighten up" before you walk in the front door to greet your significant others.

5. Be aware that stress fuels anger. Know your limits, and once you're close to the breaking point, institute stress management strategies. If you're highly stressed at work, cut yourself some slack at home (and vice versa). Cry, laugh, exercise, play, pray. At the end of a "shift from hell," slip into a darkened movie theater and transport yourself to another place and time. Take a mini-vacation by getting out postcards or souvenirs from your favorite vacation place and flying off to that place—in your imagination—for a few minutes. And avoid stress carriers, those gloomy people who consistently drag us down with their pessimism.

6. Avoid useless, no-win arguments. If possible, simply exit gracefully. Why let yourself get involved in heated discussions of abortion, politics, religion, or other value-laden topics? If you are ultimately drawn into the argument, try to find some areas of agreement to emphasize: "There are good points on both sides of this issue"; "We're both right"; "We both want the same thing." Avoid the impulse to try to win. You can't.

7. Avoid environmental stimuli and interpersonal situations that you know from past experience will "push your button." If it drives you up the wall to listen to Joann's nonstop monologue at lunch, go to lunch with Karen instead. If you fume every time you walk past Adrian's messy office, go down the other corridor so you won't have to look at it. If every board meeting of an organization is spent in fruitless bickering, resign from the board and lend your talents to other groups.

8. Work on anger issues left over from your family of origin, your divorce, or other past events. Chronic, festering anger can be devastating to your physical and mental health. Find a counselor who will help you let go of old anger (and see Chapter 8 for plenty of good self-help strategies). Psychologist Jack Kornfield (1993) tells of a man who visualized his anger as enormous—like a bomb, a nuclear explosion. When instructed to let his anger open as much as needed, the man imagined that it burned up the whole universe. Kornfield relates,

> *The whole universe became dark and dead and full of ashes. A great fear arose in him. He felt that for a long time much of his life had been dead; now the deadness felt stronger, as if his life would be that way forever. I suggested that he let the deadness and ashes fill the universe forever and see what would happen. . . . Then, to his amazement, there came a green light far off in the distance. . . . It*

was a new planet being born, with oceans, green plants, and young children. Seeing this he realized that even the greatness of his own pain had an end. The anger and frustration that had been there so long began to lose its power over him and an inevitable renewal began to take place. (Kornfield, 1993, pp. 115–116)

9. Reward yourself for trying new anger behaviors. Rewards are essential in learning and maintaining any new skills. Buy a new CD, browse in a bookstore, or go to the beach. Spend time with people who support the changes you are making. Their affirmation can be immensely valuable to the success of your behavior change project. Contact your local mental health center or university to find anger management or assertiveness groups. I regularly conduct such groups in my community. The support that I see the group members giving to each other is at least as valuable as my cheerleading for their efforts—maybe more valuable. This is a great segue to Part Two of the book, which is all about making connections with others.

II

Connecting
With Others

5

Opening Dialogue With Colleagues

> Man is but a network of relationships,
> and these alone matter to him.
>
> Maurice Merleau-Ponty

If we accept Merleau-Ponty's premise, and I imagine that most of us do, it logically follows that the healing we need in our profession cannot be accomplished by each of us working on our anger management tactics in isolation. Healing takes place in relationships, and this chapter focuses on our relationships with colleagues—other nurses, supervisors, and physicians. There is disharmony in all of our collegial relationships, as so vividly shown in the nurses' words in Chapter 1.

We work in conflict-prone organizations. According to Stokols (1992), conflict-prone organizations are characterized by the presence of rigid ideologies, nonparticipatory organizational processes, absence of shared goals, existence of competitive coalitions, and prospects of unemployment stemming from economic changes. Nurses in many diverse practice areas will recognize these qualities in their place of employment and readily understand why the place is rife with conflict. Conflict erupts even during stable periods, because it is inevitable when humans interact. But it is especially evident during times of rapid environmental and social change such as this.

WOUNDING ONE ANOTHER WITH WORDS

One of the most disturbing aspects of our research data on nurses' anger is the vehemence of their anger at each other. This nurse-to-nurse anger is not healthy anger. Words taken right from our interview transcripts include faultfinding, bickering, backbiting, needling, snapping, and cutting. These hurtful behaviors are manifestations of a phenomenon called horizontal violence, or horizontal hostility, in the literature. I have known about this destructive phenomenon—and experienced it, of course—over the 40 years that I have been in nursing. Horizontal hostility is a characteristic of oppressed groups who fight among each other because they cannot vent anger at their superiors. Throughout the history of modern nursing, physicians, supervisors, and hospital administrators have held the power over nurses. Today, despite many notable advances in the profession, the majority of nurses still work in hospitals or other facilities where there is a hierarchical system, with one or more levels of personnel above them. And they still vent their hostility horizontally toward their own peers. It's actually getting worse in these difficult times. In an organizational climate of fear, when workers do not know when—or if—they too may be laid off or lose their jobs, horizontal hostility increases. One vice president of nursing at a university hospital reported a dramatic increase in employee complaints about other employees; 80% of these complaints were false allegations made out of spite and fear (Curtin, 1995). There seems to be a grain of truth in the old cliché: *In times of fear, nurses put their wagons in a circle—but start firing at each other.*

When the "firing" is overt, as in a verbal blast or sarcastic put-down by a colleague, it may be easier to deal with than when it is an ambush or covert sniper fire. It's harder to identify a hidden sniper who is carrying tales to management or spreading malicious gossip. It's also hard to defend yourself when you don't know exactly what is being said. I was certainly caught off guard a few years ago when colleagues of mine went behind my back to the director of the educational institution where I taught at the time. I was serving on a committee that was spinning its wheels. I grew weary of unproductive debate and suggested that a small task force or subcommittee be appointed to delve into the matter and bring recommendations back to the larger group. No one voiced an objection to this suggestion, and the meeting was adjourned shortly thereafter. To my astonishment, the next day I was summoned to the office of the director. I was informed that the other committee members thought that I was "rude," and that I had hurt their feelings. My action was perceived as cutting off debate prematurely. Rather than forthrightly saying to me, "No, appointing a task force is not the way to go," members of the committee had gone to the director to complain. The director warned me to be more careful in the future.

Examples of the more subtle forms of horizontal hostility abounded in our research data:

I tend to draw back from her and give her a lot of the cold shoulder.

I am a female Southerner, trained from birth to be passive-aggressive. You can cut them, but don't let them know they're bleeding until they look down and see it.

Helen Campbell spoke of "closet things" and coworkers "hugging you and stabbing you at the same time." She experienced no hostility from these coworkers when she was an LPN, but when she returned to the same ICU to work as a charge nurse, their attitude was different. She isn't sure whether their behavior should be attributed to racism or gender:

I've worked at this institution for 17 years. I was tolerated as long as I was an LPN. I wasn't a threat because I was on a lower level. Now I'm an RN like everybody else and I'm the only black in the ICU with eight white nurses. I've always had the ability, but now I've got the license to go with it. And now they all resent me. I didn't ask for a charge position; it was of- fered to me. There were plots. They would do deceitful things. I found out females do that anyway.

Does this horizontal hostility occur in our profession because nurses are predominantly women, "trained from birth to be passive-aggres- sive," as one of the nurses described? It is true that nursing has been viewed as "women's work," and certainly "women's work"—nurturing and caring for others—has been devalued in our society, just as women themselves have been. In a patriarchal culture women are viewed as subordinate and inferior to men, and they internalize the culture's view of them. Thus, it is difficult for women to view other women as valuable. It is also true that chilly silence, cattiness, snide memos, and other pas- sive-aggressive behaviors are pervasive in female-dominated profes- sional groups. In one recent survey, more than 75% of the female nurse respondents said they had been undermined by another woman (Briles, 1994). But it was clear from our study of male nurses that hori- zontal hostility is not confined to females. We saw many instances of it in our sample of male RNs. They too made disparaging remarks about colleagues. They too experienced frequent verbal attacks from cowork- ers. One male nurse spoke of being "wounded with words." Another said, "She purposely attacked me, embarrassing me in front of others, humiliating me, trying to make me look incompetent. I should have been more assertive. But I wasn't at that time." The devastating phenomenon of horizontal hostility does not occur just because most nurses are women. It occurs because all of us in the profession—male and female alike—have been oppressed.

Some of us deal with oppression by identifying with the oppressor. I saw an example of this recently in Tennessee. A woman who had a satisfying birth experience in the care of a nurse-midwife wrote a very positive letter to the local newspaper. Other letter writers joined in the ensuing dialogue, expressing largely favorable opinions. There was only one dissenting voice: that of an obstetric nurse. In her belligerent letter, she claimed that a woman would choose a nurse-midwife only if "there is no higher skilled person available or because they have been misinformed as to the merits of nurse-midwifery." The obstetric nurse's hostility toward her colleagues becomes even more painfully evident as she continued: "I would like to make a point of saying that over the history of legitimate obstetrical care it has not been the nurse-midwife who has made the advances in prenatal care possible for pregnant women. It has been the physicians and the vast bodies of research and development available to them." By glorifying physicians and denigrating the work of those in her own profession, this letter writer is identifying with the oppressor. It is a way of dealing with her feelings of inferiority. The obstetric nurse believes she will gain greater respect and approval by aligning herself with physicians. It is physicians, not nurse-midwives, who give "legitimate obstetrical care." She cannot even acknowledge that research is done by, or available to, nurses.

When the role of physician assistant was a new one, a number of nurses felt very special in being chosen by a particular physician to receive additional preparation and then work with him. After their transformation into what they thought was a more prestigious position, they would come to the units wearing lab coats, not uniforms, seeing the physician's patients and writing orders, signing their names with PA instead of RN. Leaving off the RN credential was a clear repudiation of their former "inferior" status as a nurse. Identification with the oppressor is also seen in nurses who align themselves with hospital associations and other groups to fight against changes in legislation being proposed by their own colleagues in the state nurses' association or board of nursing. Many have internalized the views of their hospital administrators, and they believe that "the hospital knows what's best for us." I have observed numerous examples of this over the years.

Name-calling and disparaging the competence of one's colleagues are particularly destructive manifestations of nurse-to-nurse horizontal hostility. For example, Sue Green refers to some of her colleagues in advanced practice as "dizzy Lizzies" and "bad apples": *"There are some of us who really throw piles of shit on that image because they are so incompetent or, you know, dizzy Lizzy, and I think that is a situation where one bad apple can spoil a bushel."* Carol Carter calls her charge nurse a "dingbat" and asserts that the woman is unqualified and lazy: *"She was getting paid for charge nurse. They had a body to fill the slot. They didn't care if they had a* qualified *body. . . . She was getting paid, but yet she didn't do anything. Here I'm working my behind off as a staff nurse and my other coworkers are working their behinds off and yet we had another body getting paid more salary, doing nothing."* Ron Murray related an acrimonious exchange with a "haughty" coworker who questioned his nursing knowledge: *"She got loud, sort of haughty, and I said, 'You just better stop 'cause I'm not taking this crap off of you. I don't give you crap and you're not going to give me crap. It's disrespectful."*

Not only do nurses devalue each other, they also devalue themselves. It was distressing to the members of my research team to hear so many nurses—smart and capable professionals—devaluing their own work. For example, Eve Sanders, a master's prepared nurse practitioner, referred to her work as "scut work" and "taking care of the petty things." Every nurse whom we interviewed used the word *hierarchy* and had a definite perception of where they and others belonged in the hierarchy of health care providers. Doctors held superior rank in the echelon, and there was even a hierarchical ordering within nursing itself, with critical care nursing accorded higher status than psychiatric or maternal-child nursing. Sadly, nurses who provide magnificent direct patient care every day, a vital service to humanity, put themselves down by saying things like "I'm just a staff nurse" or "I was never able to go back to school to get my bachelor's degree."

The oppression starts in nursing school for many of us. Just as Meissner (1986) proposed in her classic article, nurses *do* eat our young. Nurse educators are the first offenders. Rather than encouraging students to develop and use their personal power, many teachers are "drill sergeants" commanding obedience. In the clinical area, there is more emphasis on judging students than on assisting and supporting them. And the classroom is a place of humiliation for many. According to Meissner, "We assign unrealistic study loads and written assignments that may seem little related to their clinical activities. . . . But it's in testing and grading that we become the great gobblers of our young. We write minutiae-filled examinations that make it nearly impossible for students with excellent grades in general courses to attain similar grades in work that matters to them most—their major. Is it any wonder that many students who entered nursing with great expectations fail to thrive?" (Meissner, 1986, p. 52).

While Meissner calls the phenomenon insidious cannibalism, Jarratt (1981) proposed that faculty behavior is analogous to child abuse: "The 'we' who were being mistreated or misunderstood then, are the 'they' of today" (p. 10). Regardless of what you label it, it is clear that inhumane treatment of nursing students has been going on for a long time. Distinguished nursing scholar Jeanne Quint Benoliel was a student nurse in a diploma program from 1938 to 1941. She was 500 miles away from home, living by a strict code of rules in a dormitory next to the hospital. Even after more than 50 years, she vividly remembers how she felt when accused of stealing from a patient:

> *Fear of negligence was inculcated in us by the attitudes and actions of the faculty, who seemed to equate making mistakes with committing mortal sins. . . . I was assigned to obstetrics. I had not been there very long and had little experience or knowledge about the prepartum events to expect. I was assigned to stay with a woman of Italian background who came in on the evening shift with her husband and her mother. She had started labor while they were having dinner, and while in the hospital, she started vomiting. I think that part of what I did was to complete the admission process, but I mainly remember being in the room with the three of them and not knowing what to do to help this woman feel better. She was not easy to be with because she expressed her discomfort vocally and loudly. At some point I was relieved by someone else, and I went to the dorm to get some sleep. In the early morning hours I was awakened to take a phone call from the night supervisor, who wanted to know what I had done with the woman's valuables. The tone of her voice was accusatory. I could not remember. So I got dressed and went to the woman's room to see if I could remember anything. I looked in the bedside drawer—and lo and behold, there were her things! I reported the information to the night supervisor and then went back to my room, where I cried and cried. I was angry at being treated as though I were a criminal, but I assumed that I had to "take it" because that was the pattern of superior-subordinate relationships. . . . I remember the incident as another of those "put-down" experiences by a senior nurse.*

Research supports the continued existence of "put-down" experiences of our novice nurses. Ellis (1980) found that self-confidence and self-esteem of nursing students decreased with each subsequent year of enrollment in the nursing program. Negative interaction with instructors was identified as the most anxiety-producing aspect of clinical experience in a study of baccalaureate students conducted by Kleehammer, Hart, and Keck (1990). In a more recent study that I conducted with my colleagues Johnie Mozingo and Ellie Brooks, baccalaureate students were still saying they were "intimidated" by faculty and "drilled in front of doctors and nurses" (Mozingo, Thomas, & Brooks, 1995). These statements were typical:

> *Few instructors give encouragement and tell you when you have done a good job—you always hear the negative.*
> *It seemed as if instructors constantly looked for wrong things.*
> *Instructors give it to us good when we mess up.*

Practicing nurses interviewed by my research team provided additional evidence. One nurse recalled an instructor that obviously delighted in pouncing upon a student's inadequacies:

> *"You could hear her out at the nurses' station and somebody would say to her, 'How's everything going?' and she'd say, 'Oh, I'm just sitting here giving that student just enough rope to hang herself.'"*Another nurse told us: *"Faculty sometimes can see a student with a lot of potential and will cut a student down just to put her in her place."*

Nurse administrators and staff nurses often carry on where the faculty leave off. When the new graduates hit the workplace, their idealism is mocked and their shortcomings magnified. The failure of experienced nurses to support the new graduate was briefly mentioned in Chapter 1. Remember Bob Hayes, who was about ready to chuck it all and go back to K-Mart? Here is another poignant example from our data:

> *When I first started working here, we had a new grad who is an excellent nurse. . . . I think other nurses were jealous of her. She was a baccalaureate nurse and a lot of the nurses on my floor are not. . . . You could just see the potential in this girl. She was so good with the patients and she had a lot of energy. . . . But other nurses would never help her. It was almost like [they were] setting her up . . . to fail. . . . She told me, "I really wonder if I should be a nurse. Maybe I . . . should do something else." So I encouraged her to get off that unit. I said, "You can't let other people destroy you."*

We must stop the horizontal hostility. There is no possible winner in these destructive skirmishes with one another. Furthermore, as Theodore Roosevelt said, "There are enough targets to aim at without firing at each other." In fact, if we stay focused on fighting among ourselves, we will not have the energy to fight the bigger battles that so urgently need our attention, nor will we feel satisfied with our jobs. Group cohesion strongly influences nurses' job satisfaction (Lucas, Atwood, & Hagaman, 1993). If our profession is distinctive because of our caring, as Jean Watson, Margaret Newman, Madeleine Leininger, and others have claimed, then we must start caring for each other. We must substitute support and empathy for antagonism and mistrust.

The benefits of support are legion. The more the nurse perceives support from colleagues in the workplace, the less he or she burns out, as shown in eight studies reviewed by Duquette et al., (1994). Furthermore, as shown in another study, the beneficial effect of collegial support in preventing burnout is evident regardless of the level of job stress (Ogus, 1990). Support does not lower nurses' stress, but aids them in coping with it and adds positive need-fulfilling elements to their lives. Nurses reporting high support from coworkers also have a stronger sense of personal accomplishment than nurses reporting few sources of support (Ogus, 1990). Clearly, healing the emotional pain in nursing begins by connecting with one another.

Steps Toward Healing

1. Share yourself. I strongly believe that each of us must begin reaching out to one another. My thoughts have been influenced by Sidney Jourard's (1971) research on self-disclosure, which showed so clearly that none of us can attain health and fullest personal development unless we permit our authentic selves to be known. What does this entail? Candidly telling a coworker that you are scared or hurt. Dropping your mask of perfection or imperturbability, your defensive front, and permitting yourself to be vulnerable and real. Schopenhauer compares humans to porcupines that are trying to huddle together on a cold night to get warm. The closer they get to each other for warmth, the more they hurt each other with their sharp quills. Yet even porcupines have a soft side that is not so well defended against being touched. Thus, they can turn their soft, vulnerable undersides toward each other and achieve intimacy.

2. Listen to your colleagues when they disclose their real selves and their honest opinions. I am talking about listening in a new way, engaging in dialogue that creates a culture of cooperation. Here I am drawing from the ideas of the late David Bohm (1990) about

dialogue. He envisioned diverse people coming together to listen deeply to one another and discover new ways to work (or live) together. In dialogue, individuals give consideration to views that differ substantially from their own. Dialogue proceeds at a slower pace than normal conversation because deeper levels of listening and reflection are required. Behaviors that support dialogue are (a) listening and speaking with judgment suspended, (b) respecting differences, (c) setting aside individuals' usual roles and statuses, (d) keeping a proper balance between inquiry about another's perspectives and advocacy of your own ideas, and (e) focusing on learning from one another and expanding your understanding. Hundreds of dialogue groups have formed around the world, and my dream is that nurses can become a part of this worthwhile activity. Dialogue among a team of nurses who work together is always enlightening because each nurse's view of the work situation is only a partial view. When all members of a team disclose their perspectives to one another, awareness is enlarged and creative strategies to cope with problems can be shared.

3. Make a warm, empathic response to a colleague in distress. Empathy is not a new concept to you, and you have heard many definitions of it. I like this one from Martin Buber:

> *Empathy means, if anything, to glide with one's own feeling into the dynamic structure of . . .a man, and as it were to trace it from within, understanding the formation and mobility . . .with the perception of one's own muscles; it means to "transpose" oneself over there and in there . . . (Buber, 1965, p. 97)*

There is abundant nursing literature on empathy with patients, but I found little on nurses empathizing with each other. Just as we take note of a patient's heavy sigh, slumped shoulders, or downcast eyes, resonating with his feelings of discouragement, we can likewise be more attentive to these cues about the feelings of our colleagues. We can take a moment to show concern by putting a hand on that slumped shoulder, making contact with the downcast eyes, and offering an encouraging word. It can mean so much to a colleague if you understand that things are not going well.

When working alongside someone, our own feelings can provide useful cues about what the other is feeling. While in a group working on a care plan for a patient, Wailua Brandman (1996) tells of looking across the table at another nurse and suddenly feeling as though she herself were about to cry. Brandman did not understand why she felt this way and said nothing at the time, but after the meeting the other nurse suddenly began to cry, explaining that the meeting had been difficult for her because emotions about her father's death had surfaced. In a powerful moment of empathy between colleagues, Brandman shared her experience of wanting to cry during the meeting. The two were able to talk together about grieving.

Responding with empathy is more difficult when a coworker has just put you down or maligned you. It would be so much easier to respond to horizontal hostility in a hostile fashion, delivering a nasty zinger or plotting a diabolical act of revenge. But remember that a hostile response will surely generate still more hostility. Take a moment to remind yourself that the person who put you down did so to elevate himself. Temporarily, he (or she) feels bigger and better than you. But he's not bigger and better. Inside, he's insecure. So respond to the insecurity—with empathy.

4. Make a commitment to supportive colleagueship. This does not mean that you must like everyone with whom you work, nor do I suggest that you ignore others' half-done tasks or take them on yourself. Instead, deal with anger issues promptly and honestly, as they arise, and maintain civility. Talk directly to the person you're angry with, not to others. Keep your discussion private. When the dispute is resolved, let bygones be bygones. Eschew destructive gossip. If an angry incident is still festering because you were too infuriated to constructively problem-solve at the time, commit to reconnecting with the other person within 36 hours following the episode (Plas & Hoover-Dempsey, 1988). Make a contract to notice something positive about another nurse each week and pass it on to him or her (Gropper, 1994). Congratulate colleagues who obtain promotions, certifications, and advanced degrees. Nurses yearn for the affirmation of their colleagues but seldom receive much of it.

5. Refuse to get caught up in workplace negativism. Emotions, like viruses, are highly contagious when people live or work together in close proximity. This is especially true in the noisy, crowded, hectic workplaces where health care is delivered. Angry negative coworkers evoke our own anger. Nurses may be particularly prone to "catching" others' emotions because of their training to be empathic with others' suffering. However, the acute sensitivity to feel-

ings that gives us a clinical advantage may become a disadvantage when it comes to dissipating nonproductive anger that is heating up the workplace. Research shows that women from a variety of occupations are more susceptible to emotional contagion than men are (Doherty, Orimoto, Singelis, Hatfield, & Hebb, 1995). So it may be more important for females than for males to learn how to turn down emotional arousal or leave an angry scene to preserve their equilibrium. Research comparing female and male nurses in this regard has not been conducted, however, although the male nurses we studied seemed quite affected by the negativism in their job sites. For example, Ron Murray, an oncology nurse, seemed unable to resist being dragged down by the attitudes of others:

> *You can't come to work and have a good day because everybody's in a bad mood. You just sort of get in a negative attitude too. And if you're negative, you just do what you have to do to get through the day. When I work with different people, I have a much better day.*

Ron needs to develop better resistance to the virus of negativity.

6. Be vigilant regarding disrespectful treatment of colleagues. Although it is not always possible or appropriate to directly intervene during an incident, a supportive word afterward can mean so much. Ann Smith has a colleague who is her "sounding board." In trying moments, the two meet in the locker room. Not only does Ann obtain release by talking, but also by "hug therapy" or massage: "You're tense, you sit down and rub each other's necks, pull your shoes off and let me rub your feet. . . . We do a lot of that . . . and a lot of hugs."

7. Institute a wellness day for your work group. While "mental health days" have long been advocated—and are actually permissible in some job sites—they tend to be days of solitary activities such as sleeping late and "vegging out." Far better is the approach taken by a home care team in Virginia that is responsible for 1,500 patients. As their caseload increased, the 22-member team noted increases in their stress, anger, and frustration. Two team members had to start taking antihypertensive medication. "Wellness day" was a creative approach to the stress and helped the nurses draw closer to one another. Here's what they did. Team members with various talents planned facets of the day. For example, one nurse

whose first undergraduate degree had been in music volunteered to plan an activity involving music. On a sunny October morning, the team gathered in a park with a large pavilion and fireplace. They sipped coffee and munched muffins by a roaring fire. Among the activities as the day went on were yoga, storytelling, writing songs, an imagery exercise led by a mental health nurse clinician, and an exercise involving affirmations—along with plenty of healthy food like vegetarian chili and plenty of laughter. Members of the team have this to say about their wellness day:

> *Weeks after the activity, the effects were apparent. . . . Team members expressed themselves with greater freedom and trusted their colleagues to support them. . . . We learned to recognize each other's gifts and strengths as never before. The closeness and mutual respect were reflected in how we worked with and supported each other. (Extended Services Team, 1997, p. 68)*

8. Build team spirit by socializing outside the workplace. Business has long recognized the importance of lunches, dinners, golf outings, and birthday and holiday celebrations for team-building. There is something very important about humans breaking bread together and playing together. Nurses need to give themselves permission to play more. Perhaps our workaholic ways can be traced back to the days when nurses' residences were located right next to the hospital, so that nurses mainly shuttled back and forth between the two, seldom leaving the grounds for social outings. In essence, it was a monastic existence. Even today, we seem reluctant to build time for play into our lives. Think about the last nursing conference you attended. Typically, sessions start at dawn and continue into the night, leaving virtually no free time for socializing. There is even a speaker during lunch so that no time whatsoever is wasted in "idle chitchat." What other profession so systematically deprives its members of pleasure?

I encourage you to begin connecting with your colleagues on a social basis. Some of my best memories of my staff nurse years are the zany laughter and joyous camaraderie when a group of us would go out together after work. Socializing need not be expensive; hikes and picnics cost little. If people in your agency have not mingled socially before, take the first step and invite everyone to a covered-dish brunch or supper at your home. Keep it simple. Just have fun!

9. Become involved in a support group (if you are a psych clinical specialist or have comparable training in group leadership skills, consider offering your skills to lead a group). It is important that such a group have an experienced leader, so that it does not degenerate into a moan-and-groan session. There are a number of accounts of beneficial support groups for nurses in the literature. I will cite just one example. A psychiatric nurse specialist was asked to work with nurses in a neurological intensive care unit who were experiencing conflict after a change in unit leadership. Aligned on one side of the rift were the former manager and senior nurses, some with as much as 15 years' experience, while on the other side were the new manager and newly hired nurses. The staff voted to have a support group, led by the psych nurse, for six sessions of 1 hour every other week (possibly to be extended after evaluation). Everyone understood that the group was not to be a therapy group, but a support group to facilitate better communication and more harmonious functioning of the unit. As the sessions proceeded, hidden anger and pain were discovered and processed, leading to healing for these nurses. Notably, the animosity between the old and new managers decreased, and the larger group perceived an improved ability to communicate with each other, their patients, and the physicians who admitted patients to their unit (Brandman, 1996).

The gender composition of this group was not described, but I do want to mention some dangers of all-female groups, because in some nursing settings the workforce remains all female. It is likely that the support group leader will be perceived as a maternal figure, which will activate a host of reactions within the members: fears of being engulfed by the "mother," dependency, neediness, anger, disappointment, envy, competition, and sibling rivalry among the members vying for "mother's" acceptance. Thus, complex transference and countertransference dynamics will need to be examined. It is also likely that members of the group will have trouble acknowledging their own vulnerability, trusting that support is there, and accepting others' support when it is offered. As women, they have been socialized to meet the needs of others while denying their own, and, having internalized society's low view of their worth, they do not feel deserving of the caring of others (Ewashen, 1997). Despite these mitigating factors, all-female groups can be important vehicles for fostering personal growth and meaningful connections among the members.

10. If you teach, don't engage in dean-bashing (see the excellent article by Laurel Archer Copp (1995)), and do your part to stop the intergenerational transmission of oppression that we spoke of earlier. Resolve to develop a warm, caring environment in your classroom and to convey caring when you do clinical supervision and advising. How will students learn to be caring nurses if they see no models of caring to emulate? I feel good about the classroom environment that I create with my students because it is relaxed, with plenty of encouragement to think critically, discuss, and debate. All persons are treated with respect, and all contributions to the discussion are welcomed. But I confess that I catch myself focusing on the negative when grading student papers. Because I have spent years writing and editing, my eyes go right to a misspelled word or misplaced comma. Before long, the student's paper looks like it is hemorrhaging from all of the red marks. So I revive the memory of a teacher of mine who used pens of three colors when grading: green, purple, and orange. One color was for content, one was for style and grammar problems, and one was for American Psychological Association (APA) format problems. It must have taken this teacher hours and hours to detect and mark all of the flaws. For example, each and every time that I had not left two spaces after a period when typing my paper (a violation of APA rules) this teacher marked the error. As you can imagine, it was rather overwhelming to get a paper back with all of its mistakes vividly denoted in multicolor! Remembering how I felt at that time, I try to find some positives in my student's work.

A qualitative study of student perceptions of faculty caring (Beck, 1991) provides a clear picture of what students really want and need from their teachers. Forty-seven caring experiences were described by the nursing students: 19 had occurred in an advising session, 12 in a discussion of personal problems, 8 in clinical, and 8 in the classroom. In caring interactions, the students perceive their teachers to be nonjudgmental and unhurried. Attributes of faculty caring include focusing their complete attention on the students, conveying respect, and sharing of themselves. A faculty member's time is perceived as a valuable gift to a student. After experiencing a caring interaction, the student wishes to reach out to someone else through caring. The enormity of the effect of just one caring interaction is expressed by two students:

I shall never forget that day in her office. It was truly a moment that could have changed my destiny. Because at that moment I made the decision to tough it out and see if I could make it. That was one year ago.

I get goose pimples every time I think of this beautiful experience although it happened over 2 years ago. Thank God she listened, as all nurses should listen, not to the words or what happened but to the pain that was pouring from the heart. And because she did that, I am a happy, healthy, productive, and worthwhile human today. (Beck, 1991, p. 18)

RESOLVING CONFLICT WITH SUPERVISORS

For too long, too many nurse leaders have been much like "drum majorettes" who never look behind to see if anyone is following. It is time for nurse leaders to put down their "sequined batons" and rejoin the ranks of the marchers. (Sullivan & Deane, 1994, p. 8)

Anger at their leaders (head nurses, supervisors, clinical directors, deans) was common in our interview data from nurses. What made nurses angry was leader behavior they perceived as authoritarian, faultfinding, and uncaring. Bob Hayes, who has left ICU for home health, described several humiliating episodes of being castigated by managers he described as "rigid." His description of one such episode is illustrative:

Her body language was that of a smart ass. She was shaking her head, batting her eyes. And she had that smirky look on her face. I don't like that at all. It was just a disrespectful look. And when you do that you're not going to get positive results. You're not going to get a change. What you're going to get is a counter reaction. I was feeling rage.

Ann Smith, a labor and delivery nurse, had a manager who listened but did nothing. Ann was both frustrated and hurt by her manager's behavior. When she went to the manager with concerns about an unsafe staffing pattern, this is what happened:

She uses a lot of psychological terms: "I hear where you're coming from. I understand what you're saying." And then I get the feeling that she puts it in her back pocket and goes. . . . It's frustrating to me that the person that's directly over me and directly controls what happens in my surroundings is out of touch with what's going on with me and the people I'm working with. This is a unit-wide complaint. It's not isolated incidents. It's a long-term, day-after-day problem.

Joy Carpenter, another obstetric nurse, reported feeling a complete lack of support from her supervisor:

The minute I needed something, the supervisor would leave the floor. It was almost like the minute I said, "I need to see you," she would leave.

Ron Murray, an oncology staff nurse, viewed management as taking from him rather than assisting him to get what he needs to perform his job according to his standards:

They're always cutting this, cutting that, cutting staff. . . . I feel like I have certain standards that I should be able to keep, and when they cut staff then I'm not able to keep those standards.

Linda Harvey, a med-surg nurse, told us of experiences when managers sabotaged her. Clearly she has begun to view them as the enemy:

I have never seen where they will be your advocate. . . . Nurse administrators are no longer nurses. They have totally lost sight of the nursing side. I don't ever see it where they're really on the side of the nurse. They're loyal to the other side. And you shouldn't be at sides or at war.

Understandably, hostility builds over time when managers consistently fail to display effective leadership behavior. Social gatherings of nurses who work together are often dominated by sharing of fantasies about ways to get rid of their witchy manager: burning her at the stake, or perhaps in hot oil. In an imagery exercise in a workshop I conducted, one nurse fantasized taking the door off the closet and putting her head nurse's desk in there, behind the door. With glee, she imagined the head nurse shrieking, "It's too dark; I can't see!"

While the grievances of nurses like Bob and Ann and Joy and Ron appear to be legitimate, another dynamic is at work in some of the animosity that staff nurses feel toward their supervisors. Davies (1995) observed that "nurses have long reserved their most withering contempt for their colleagues who move up the managerial ladder, seemingly leaving real nursing for pay and power, especially when their presence in these elevated posts seems to offer little support and resourcing in the clinical setting" (p. 8). We've all heard scuttlebutt in the cafeteria about those who have "sold out to the enemy," shedding their uniforms for designer duds and leaving their poor colleagues trapped in the trenches. When the supervisor is female, as is often the case, much of this hostility toward nursing leaders can be attributed to the same devaluing transferences seen in other predominantly female groups (Ewashen, 1996). The leader is expected to be an all-perfect "mother" who will sense their needs and nurture them. Nurses are looking to the leader more so for emotional support than for decision-making. Since the ideal of a perfect, ever-nurturing mother is impossible to achieve, nurses are often disappointed in their leaders, denigrating them and colluding to prove that they are incompetent. The group culture becomes one of discouragement and anger. Subgroups may form and internal warfare may begin. Barritt (1984) used the term *emotional nepotism* to describe the cliques that form, based on emotional ties of some of the workers to one another. Being in a clique may result in favored treatment (holidays off, raises, promotions, new computers, office furniture, whatever the distributable "goodies" are), while the outsiders fume at the inequities, file grievances, and take other measures to fight back. During the infighting among the workers, scapegoats may be targeted, energy evaporates in fruitless conflict, and productivity of the unit declines. Does this sound familiar to you? It certainly does to me. I have experienced this whole destructive scenario in more than one female work group during my career.

Women distrust powerful women. They have dared to stand out from the rest. That is not looked on kindly in oppressed groups. When I was growing up in Memphis, my friends referred to such individuals as "uppity." From childhood, girls learn that their peers will disapprove if they are too self-confident or aggressive. Many women who have achieved prominence in nursing have endured considerable horizontal hostility from colleagues. Not long ago, I was reading about Loretta Ford, who developed the first program for nurse practitioners. Her colleagues at the university heaped abuse upon her, and some groups even wanted to excommunicate her from membership (Fondiller, 1995). Why does this behavior occur? After 10 years of the women's movement, novelist Margaret Atwood commented:

> *We like to think that some of the old stereotypes are fading, but 10 years is not a very long time in the history of the world, and I can tell you from experience that the old familiar images, the old icons, have merely gone underground, and not far at that. We still think of a powerful man as a born leader and a powerful woman as an anomaly, a potentially dangerous anomaly; there is something subversive about such women, even when they*

take care to be good role models. They cannot have come by their power nat-
urally, it is felt. They must have got it from somewhere. (Atwood, cited in
Eisenstein, 1988)

We still do not trust or feel comfortable with women leaders. Linda's
view, cited above, of "sides" who are "at war" conjures up the image of
adversaries in perpetual and irreconcilable combat.

Conflict with supervisory personnel contributes to nursing turnover
and even to departure from the profession. In a survey of more than
1,000 nurses across the nation, Cox (1991) found that the greater the
conflict between nurses and their administrators (both the nursing administrators and the top-level administrators), the more likely nurses
were to resign their positions. Public health nurse Sarah Prentiss, whom
you met in Chapter 2, burned out after 10 years and left the field. Although her demanding, unsympathetic supervisor was not the only
cause of her disillusionment with nursing, Sarah believes that the supervisor's behavior exacerbated her situation. Sarah related, "She did-
n't understand the frustration. She was in her office, and she just had
unrealistic expectations for the staff. She'd say, 'Oh, come on, try this,
go back and try this.'And I'd say, 'No, we've tried that.' She just had no
idea" (Cherniss, 1995, p. 72). Unlike Sarah Prentiss, Rebecca Simpson
remained in her public health position. But after her relationship with
her supervisor soured, she felt that her initiative and creativity declined.
When she proposed innovative solutions to a problem, they were not
well received. Eventually, her self-esteem was affected: "I started not
feeling very good about myself, which I think, probably sometimes
came across in my work. . . . I would have liked to have avoided the
whole mess because that was not good for me, as far as my confidence
goes, and self-image, and everything" (Cherniss, 1995, p. 140).

What is the manager's view of all of this? Our study participants
made it clear that being a manager is no picnic. Lisa Thompson, a clinical director interviewed by our research team, is weary of the competitiveness among her staff and sees her job as "continually in this
sandwich of making peace with all." She also arbitrates between the
staff nurses and physicians, with the physicians "not willing to give an
inch, not an inch, in many, many situations." Although she speaks
warmly of most of the staff she supervises, she has difficulty with some of
them who see nursing as "a job to make money and go home and pay
the bills and cook supper. It's more than that. I guess I'm idealistic, but
people need to see it as more than that. I wish they would move on. And
it's hard for me not to tell them just exactly that."

Greg James echoed Lisa's frustration about having to supervise nurses who "don't realize that they are burned out and that they need a change. And they won't broaden their horizons." Tom Parker spoke of dealing with a passive-aggressive staff member who was a chronic problem. He recalled a particularly infuriating episode when the nurse did not like his patient assignment and set off a chain reaction on the unit:

He was messing up the assignments of several other people. The others were getting angry and I was getting flak from that. I had tried to be as fair as I could with everyone. I asked everyone to take a turn in helping with this particular area so that I wasn't putting it off on any one person. His attitude angered me. I had been getting a lot of resistance from this person for a long time.

Sally Jones, a head nurse of surgery, felt that staff nurses do not understand her tremendous management responsibilities:

In their view, when you're sitting behind a desk it's not "real nursing," but I'm responsible for interviewing, hiring, firing, payroll, time and attendance, seeing that policies and procedures are carried out, and when physicians have a problem they come to me. . . . I feel like people use me, I feel like everything's being dumped on my shoulders. . . . I feel overwhelmed. I guess you don't really know who to talk to.

Greg quit management after a year:

As a manager in a hospital today it's very difficult. There is no extra money. There are no incentives. There's nothing more you can give your staff. You only have a limited supply of money and positions, and the nurse-patient ratio is getting worse and worse every day. As a manager, you listen to the venting. You get to hear all the problems all day long. If you don't have a person to vent to, you bottle it up. It just finally got to me and I decided to do something totally different.

As you can see from our interview data, middle managers and executives are frustrated, isolated, and lonely. As Lisa put it, "I will honestly say that I feel pretty much out on a limb most of the time." The work of nurse managers mandates time-consuming meetings with nonnurses who do not understand the problems they are grappling with. Their support network can be pretty thin or nonexistent. Consequently, there are few outlets for their own anger and fear. They have little opportunity to obtain constructive feedback from peers. It can be hard for a new manager to find a comfortable style. If the manager is female, she may find herself in the damned-if-you-do-damned-if-you-don't double bind that snares women in positions of authority. The conflicting advice given by male senators to their female colleagues is a good example. Senator Barbara Mikulski was advised to soften her hard-hitting style, while Senator Nancy Kassebaum was urged to be firmer and more assertive (Tannen, 1994).

What supervisory personnel *think* they are doing may not be what staff nurses are perceiving. Perceptions of staff nurses and nurse managers regarding the type of leadership in their agencies differed significantly in the study by Cox (1991). Staff nurses said the usual type of leadership was "autocratic," while nurse managers viewed it as "participative." Ashley (1976) observed that nurses in leadership positions are least effective in the areas of interpersonal relations and communicating with other nurses. Because they have not cultivated a power base or built consensus among the nurses they are supposed to be leading, they make their decisions in isolation. Hence, they are perceived as autocratic.

As you can see, there are two polarized views of "we" vs. "they." Let's work toward dropping "they" and just becoming "we." The bottom line is that nurses are all colleagues: head nurses and their staffs, deans of nursing and their faculties, coordinators and those whose work they coordinate. Current trends such as flattening of hierarchical levels, decentralization of decision-making, and shared governance should help to reduce the polarization. Clearly, there is a crying need in our profession for the development of less antagonistic, more supportive relationships between managers and their staffs. We must learn to get along better. The future of nursing depends on it. If you are a nurse manager, here are some things you can do to help smooth the waters.

WHAT MANAGERS CAN DO TO IMPROVE RELATIONSHIPS WITH STAFF

1. Conveying support to your staff must be the number one priority. This does not mean that you are going to be an all-nurturing mother, an impossible undertaking. But try to imagine, from the staff nurse's point of view, how it would feel to get a response to your call for help like that made by the sarcastic supervisor quoted in Chapter 1: "Well, where do you think I'm going to get these nurses, cut out paper dolls?" Even if the supervisor had no one to

send, there are a number of responses that would have indicated support: "I'll see what I can do. If nothing else, I'll come up myself and help you for a little while," or "I know it's rough, but the rest of the place is crazy too. I just don't have a soul, but as soon as I put out these fires down here in the ER, I'll be up."

Linda Harvey defined a supportive manager as someone who "doesn't always agree with you but who will be there even if you make a mistake." She recalled a situation in which she called her head nurse at home after she had a telephone altercation with a physician:

> *I was real lucky because this happened to be a supportive head nurse, and that is something you do not have very often; it is almost un-heard of. In fact, out of all the places I've lived and worked, she stands out in my mind. She reamed the doctor out for his behavior to-ward me. What happened is, the patient ended up coding and being intubated. Had the doctor come in, that may have been prevented.*

Research data on the importance of supervisor support is plentiful. In a survey of 8,023 RNs, what the nurses wanted most was support from nursing management ("Nursing Shortage Poll Report," 1988). High supervisor support has been shown to aid nurses in coping with negative aspects of their jobs (Constable & Russell, 1986). And a recent meta-analysis that aggregated the data from 48 studies, with a total of 15,048 nurse participants, revealed that good communication with supervisors was a significant predictor of job satisfaction (Blegen, 1993).

2. Realize that you, by virtue of your leadership position, are sometimes going to be the "lightning rod" for staff anger in your facility. This can be extremely threatening and anxiety-producing. It is understandable that your initial impulse may be to avoid the angry person or group. Feeling inadequate to cope with the anger, you may postpone attending to it. However, as pointed out by Morath, Casey, and Covert (1985), "Anger that is not dealt with results in lost opportunities for learning and growth; problems are unidentified and unresolved, staff relations are painful, trust erodes, and eventually patient care deteriorates" (p. 45). It is important that you listen to the angry individual in a setting of privacy and confidentiality, without defensiveness or retaliation. Let the nurse have his or her say. Ascertain if there are substantive issues that need your attention. Then consider alternative responses. If the nurse's

anger is irrational or disproportionate to the situation, try the approach of noted leader Rosalee Yeaworth:

> *While I was dean, a member of my administrative team sent very excoriating memorandums whenever she disagreed with something I did or didn't do. Taken by surprise the first time or two this happened, I became angry that she hadn't come to discuss the concerns face-to-face. I sent a rather heated response, trying to explain and defend my reasoning. She, in turn, sent an even more scathing memorandum, and it was obvious that the written word was escalating the angry feelings. I had my secretary arrange an appointment for us to meet face-to-face, and we were able to discuss matters quite civilly. I was surprised that she didn't seem nearly as angry as the memo seemed to indicate. She admitted that sitting down and writing such a memo served as a catharsis and made her feel much better. During the 12 or so years that we worked together, she continued periodically to send me very angry memorandums, but after my initial experience, I would read them, take a few deep breaths, and put them under my "to do" pile. I would wait a few days until we both had cooled off, and I perhaps had gathered more information, then arranged for a face-to-face meeting. Despite these periodic episodes, we were able to work together, have some good accomplishments, retain respect for each other's perspectives, and, I believe, remain friends.*

3. Rein in your own anger. Managers who react in a volatile fashion add to the stress in the work environment and set a poor example for those under their supervision. Remember that the short-term effects of anger outbursts may seem positive (anger does get people's attention), but staff morale and productivity will decline over the long term. Your anger outbursts can also lead to high turnover of staff. Trust and respect of staff are earned by demonstrations of level-headed, consistent behavior.

4. Be alert to troubled nurses who need help. Behaviors such as extreme anger, subversive activities, decreased productivity, or increased absenteeism indicate a need for intervention. One angry, negative individual can cause tremendous havoc in a work site. Jane Halsey, a director of nursing services in Washington D.C., has discovered that in many cases these nurses are plagued by home or personal problems such as marital strife, financial crisis, illness or death in the nurse's family, or inability to conceive a child. Although the old adage advises "leaving your troubles on the door-

step" when you come to work, it is difficult to compartmentalize your life, particularly when strong emotions are involved. Halsey (1985) provided the following guidelines for dealing with the troubled nurse:

> Begin by sitting down with the nurse and having a one-to-one fact-finding session.
>
> Present facts about the unacceptable behavior.
>
> Ascertain if there are training needs or work environment problems.
>
> If personal problems surface, do not suggest a solution.
>
> Listen, allow the nurse to express feelings.
>
> Consider alterations in work hours or work unit.
>
> Refer the nurse to a counselor. If the work performance is in need of immediate improvement so that the nurse will not be terminated, the referral can be mandatory, and the counselor can be asked to verify kept appointments.
>
> Make plans for follow-up sessions at specific intervals. Give positive reinforcement for improvements in attitude and work performance.

5. Model individuation for your staff despite group pressure to be "one of us" (McWilliams & Stein, 1987, p. 149). If you are a female, break out of the protective mother role. Be a mentor, not a mother. Deal with staff dependency, envy, and competition. In a largely female professional group, the opportunities for female nurses to replay difficulties of separating from mother, individuating, and satisfying dependency needs are endless. But in the replaying, corrective learning experiences can take place: You as a new kind of mother-authority figure can mentor younger nurses to grow in self-definition and autonomy (Ruiz, 1988).

6. Learn all you can about transformational leadership. Take courses, attend continuing education conferences, consider pursuit of graduate preparation in nursing administration. Too often, the goal of nursing managers is to control. While managers control an enterprise, leaders know how to bring out the best in people and respond quickly to change (Naisbett & Aburdene, 1990). Early views of leadership emphasized motivating workers to do tasks and rewarding them with "carrots" for compliance instead of punishing them with "sticks." While positive reinforcement is undoubtedly preferable to the alternative, Levinson (1980) pointed out

that even if the leader uses carrots instead of sticks, the follower will continue to feel like a jackass. Transformational leadership is more effective and satisfying than contingent rewarding. Supporting evidence, in the form of field studies, interviews, case histories, and laboratory investigations, has been gathered around the world (Bass, 1997). So nowadays, the prevailing paradigm is transformational leadership, which motivates followers to go beyond their own self-interests for the good of the group or organization. Transformational leaders inspire their staffs to do more than they originally expected to do (Burns, 1978). They are admired as role models, generating pride and loyalty.

What are the characteristics of a transformational leader? According to the research literature, which has been summarized by Bass (1997), such a leader

- takes stands on difficult issues and displays conviction
- articulates an optimistic, appealing vision of the future
- inspires and challenges followers with high standards
- provides encouragement for what needs to be done
- stimulates in others new perspectives and ways of doing things
- deals with others as individuals, considering their needs and abilities
- listens attentively, advises, teaches, and coaches

Florence Nightingale would surely be categorized as a transformational leader. Why has our profession produced only one Nightingale? What are we doing in schools of nursing, employing agencies, and professional organizations to prepare the next generation of leaders? Nurses are hungry for transformational leaders and the organizational climates that they create. We want role models whom we can trust and emulate. Yes, we have some effective leaders and managers in nursing, but we need more. In the meantime, we can't leave all the work of reconciliation to our managers. We must make some efforts to connect more effectively with them too. Here are some tips for doing so:

WHAT STAFF CAN DO TO IMPROVE
RELATIONSHIPS WITH MANAGERS

1. Tell your manager what you want or need. Contrary to popular assumption, managers cannot read minds. Recall Fran (Chapter 3),

who expected her supervisor to come to her rescue, even though she had not asked for help. Fran—and the patients on her unit—would have been much better off if she had made an assertive request for more personnel. When you make a request, be clear and direct. Don't give your manager the impression that you're being critical. Express your appreciation for the opportunity to voice your concerns.

2. When you have a burning grievance, don't strike while the iron is red hot. Cool down, strategize, then go to the manager or supervisor. State the issue or problem in very specific terms. For example, "I am angry that I have been changed to night shift for the next month." Discuss only one problem at a time; don't bring up a laundry list of old anger-provoking incidents. Listen carefully to your manager's response. Restate it to make sure you understood exactly what was said: "If I understood correctly, you're saying that you see no alternative but for me to work nights while John is away." Avoid making any inferences or asking accusatory questions ("Why wasn't Karen asked to pull graveyard shift? Karen always gets treated with kid gloves"). Brainstorm to come up with alternative solutions. Be willing to accept a compromise. After all, *somebody* has to work nights. Maybe you can take part of the shifts in John's absence, while Karen will be asked to do the rest of them.

3. Be a team player. If you are a woman in your 30s or older, you probably didn't have an opportunity to play team sports when you were growing up. Certain concepts, such as loyalty to the team, aren't second nature to you. Men traditionally have had an advantage here. Critique your own behavior, your interaction not only with the "coach," but also with the other members of the team. Are your actions promoting success of the work team or undermining it? Remember that the outcome of leadership rests ultimately with the followers.

4. Give your manager some support. It's a tough job. Remember the metaphor of the crab bucket: You do not need to put a lid on a bucket of crabs because when one crab gets to the top, the others will pull it down (Hagberg, 1984). Do you really want to pull your manager down? When you feel critical of your manager, remind yourself that you do not have access to all of the information that he or she has. Imagine what it would be like to endure all the crabs pulling at you. When is the last time you told your manager that he or she is doing a good job? What could you do to make that job a bit easier?

RESOLVING CONFLICT WITH PHYSICIANS

Although their education, training, and traditions differ, physicians and nurses share a common commitment to patient well-being. Because of this commitment, it makes good sense for physicians and nurses to consider themselves colleagues. A more collegial, unified relationship between nurses and physicians will improve patient care . . . (Gianakos, 1997, p. 57).

These words, taken from a recent article in *Nursing Outlook*, were written by a physician, who went on to say that he viewed collegiality as a moral imperative. He asserted that "good patient care requires that physicians and nurses work together in a collaborative and respectful manner" (Gianakos, 1997, p. 57). I couldn't agree more. Nurses told my research team that this collegial relationship is exactly what they want. In too many situations, however, this is an ideal yet to be achieved. As you will recall from Chapter 1, disrespectful treatment by physicians provoked deep anger in nurses. Our study participants described criticism, attacks, tirades, and baseless accusations. They said doctors used them as "scapegoats" and "whipping posts." They experienced being "lambasted," "thrashed," "picked on," "belittled," and "lectured." When there were observers to these incidents, such as their peers or patients, the humiliation was especially galling to the nurses. The story related to our research team by Mike Evans, an ICU/CCU nurse whom you met in Chapter 1, is illustrative of a number of common themes, including outrage, helplessness, a sense of betrayal, and ultimately a severed relationship:

There was a cardiac surgeon. I tried to beep him several times during the night to call him some blood gases. He wouldn't return my call, and I ended up having to call his partner. His partner gave me orders not to wean the patient any further until morning. I knew the first surgeon would be angry about that when he came in and saw that the patient hadn't been weaned, so I went ahead and weaned him . . . to where he could have been extubated shortly after the surgeon saw him in the morning.

The first physician came in the next morning and was extremely angry, not that I had weaned the patient but that I didn't have him already extubated, even though I had orders from his partner not to wean him at all. . . . He just thrashed me verbally in front of my peers. . . . demanded to see the supervisor and tried to get me fired. . . . My supervisor wanted to know why I didn't have him weaned further. I said, "Well, I had orders not to wean him at all."

When asked by the interviewer how he felt, Mike expressed outrage at the physician's behavior:

His outburst was totally unprofessional and unwarranted. . . . What he was angry about was totally, totally ludicrous. . . . I really had no idea what set him off . . . As he was thrashing me, his partner came in and said, "I told Mike not to wean him further at all." The second surgeon was supportive of me. . . . I guess it was trying to please the first surgeon that got me in trouble.

Mike went on to reveal that he had formerly felt pride in his relationship of mutual respect with the cardiac surgeon. He now considers the relationship severed:

He has traditionally liked me taking care of his patients. That's what's really bewildering to me. . . . Because I respected him, I wanted him to respect me. I wanted to have that good relationship. I tried so hard to please him, but there was no pleasing him. I'm sorry our relationship ended the way it did.

Much of the physician behavior described by our study participants can be correctly classified as verbal abuse. Make no mistake that verbal abuse is a means of holding power over other people. It is grossly inhumane and unprofessional behavior. Unfortunately, quite a lot of it is occurring: Two recent investigations reveal a high incidence of abusive behavior by physicians. Ninety percent of a sample of randomly selected staff nurses in Missouri said they had experienced verbal abuse by physicians during the past year (Manderino & Berkey, 1995). Emotional reactions reported by the nurses included anger, frustration, and disgust. Long-term effects included both negative relationship with the offending doctor and decreased job satisfaction. In another study, 64% of the nurses reported verbal abuse from a physician at least once every 2 or 3 months, and 30% experienced sexual propositions, touches, or insults, with young, white women reporting the highest incidence of sexual abuse. Twenty-three percent of the sample had had at least one experience with a physician in which their physical person was threatened, most often by having an object thrown at them. Most abusive interactions with doctors took place at the nursing station or on the ward; 39% occurred with the patient present. There were adverse consequences for patient care: When doctors acquired a reputation for tantrums, some nurses hesitated to call them about a patient or make suggestions about the patient's care (Diaz & McMillin, 1991). It should be noted that our study (Brooks et al., 1996) seems to be the first that has included male nurses; the previous studies sampled only females. Further study of the abuse received by men is warranted.

What do nurses do when these attacks occur? At the moment of the abusive treatment, the nurse may feel thrown off balance. The behavior of the physician may be completely unexpected and incomprehensible, as several nurses in our study related. Bewildered, they struggled to formulate a rational explanation for the abusive attack. They wondered if they could have said or done something differently to escape the attack. It is a mistake to try to analyze abusive behavior because it is irrational. How then should you cope with it?

Coping With Physician Abuse

Research shows that factors such as self-esteem and assertiveness contribute most to nurses' ability to cope with verbal abuse (Cox, 1991). Elsewhere in the book are detailed discussions of both of these topics. For now, here are some recommendations about what to do if you are being verbally abused by a physician (these are applicable to other abusive situations as well):

1. You are not responsible for the abuse and need not defend yourself. No matter what alleged acts of omission or commission provoked the physician, you do not deserve to be threatened, yelled at, or insulted.
2. Set firm limits on the abusive behavior by forcefully saying, "Stop that" or "Don't talk to me that way!" Make it clear that the behavior is unacceptable and you will not tolerate it. Stand tall and make direct eye contact.
3. Ask colleagues to support you. In some institutions, nurses agree to call a special kind of "code" when a colleague is being abused: All nurses on the unit come to stand with the nurse in support. Work together to develop effective sanctions and grievance procedures.
4. Be aware that you can leave an abusive situation. If the physician is having a tirade, you do not have to remain and endure it. Never allow a physician to abuse you verbally in front of a patient. This is upsetting to the patient and may diminish his or her respect for both the doctor and you.

Not only must physician abuse be eradicated, but we must come to understand obstacles to more collegial relationships. What are some of them?

Understanding Obstacles to Collegiality

There is a substantial amount of literature on the nurse-physician relationship, which has been hierarchical rather than collegial since the time of Nightingale. Some say we nurses have looked to male physicians as our father figures just as we have looked to female supervisors as our mother figures. If we are in a childlike posture with regard to doctors, we can hardly be collegial. I won't attempt to summarize all of this literature here, but let's examine a few of the obstacles to physician-nurse collegiality that have been identified. Beatrice and Philip Kalisch (1977) began their analysis by taking us back to the "awe" with which nurses viewed physicians, as shown in this 1896 poem:

> Nurses moving quietly,
> Voices hushed in awe,
> All things silent waiting,
> Obedient to the law
> That we have heard so often,
> But I'll repeat once more:
> "All things must be in order
> When Doctor's on the floor."
>
> (from *Trained Nurse Hospital Review,* 1896,
> cited in Kalisch & Kalisch, 1977)

I find that this poem accurately depicts the deference of nurses to physicians when I was a student nurse. To inculcate proper subservience, nursing schools were tightly run institutions. Our instructors taught us to stand when a doctor entered the nurse's station, to give up our seat if the doctor needed one, and to hover nearby throughout the doctor's stay on the unit. The nurse walked behind the doctor as he made rounds, carrying the charts, answering his questions, and jotting down his verbal orders. A good little handmaiden would even serve him. coffee.

I am deliberately saying "he" as I refer to doctors, because at that time most of them were men, and most of us nurses were women. Ashley (1976) described the hospital as a "household," where nurses were responsible for meeting needs of all members of the "family," from patients to physicians. From its beginning as a modern profession, medicine systematically excluded women, remaining a male-dominated field until the relatively recent inroads of larger numbers of women. Nursing was "women's work," as clearly articulated in the literature of the early 1900s: "Women are peculiarly fitted for the onerous task of patiently and skillfully caring for the patient in faithful obedience to the physician's orders. Ability to care for the helpless is women's distinctive nature. Nursing is mothering. Grownup folks when very sick are all babies" (cited by Eisenstein, 1988, p. 104). Duplicated in the health care setting was the same gendered world that existed outside, in which males took charge and led and women respectfully followed. I think that the doctor-nurse relationship was even more autocratic than other male-female relationships because the doctor's self-concept of omnipotence exceeded the average male's estimate of himself.

Hans Mauksch once captured the difference between physician education and nursing education in two succinct sentences: "Medicine presents every new fact to its student with a philosophy that goes like this: 'Here's another piece of knowledge that will make you more powerful.' Nursing presents its lore with a different tone: 'Here's another piece of knowledge. Don't you dare forget it, or you may end up hurting someone'" (Mauksch, cited in Barnum, 1989). Consequently, throughout the process of his education, the physician is acquiring a sense of power. The nurse, in contrast, is becoming more intimidated and fearful.

The classic study by Erving Goffman (1967) delineated many of the subtle, nonverbal behaviors that maintained the power inequalities of the hospital milieu. For example, Goffman pointed out that doctors frequently called nurses by their first names, while nurses were expected to address physicians as "Dr. _____." Doctors had the privilege of swearing, sitting in undignified positions, and initiating joking and bantering with nurses and other underlings, while such behaviors were unacceptable for nurses. More recent examples of power inequality were observed by journalists Bernice Buresh and Suzanne Gordon (1996). They watched as a nurse who needed to speak to a physician about a patient stood quietly beside him while he talked to another physician. The two doctors continued to talk, never acknowledging the nurse's presence. Eventually, the nurse shrugged and walked away. Later, one of the doctors who had ignored the nurse barged into the nurses' station, firing questions rapidly. The nurses, despite the rudeness of his interruption, immediately stopped their own work and gave him the information he needed. In both instances, the doctors made it clear that their needs took precedence over anything a nurse might want to communicate or do. A nurse's work is interruptible, theirs is not.

Physicians have sought to maintain their paternalistic dominance over nursing in a number of ways. For example, at the turn of the century nurses were forbidden to read the medical histories of patients, and numbers rather than drug names were placed on drug bottles (Lovell, 1988). Doctors have consistently opposed nurses becoming better educated. The American Medical Association (AMA) opposed federal aid to nursing and successfully blocked bills that would have enabled the profession to upgrade educational levels. In many states, physicians sat on boards of nursing, meddling in the governance of nursing practice. One physician, writing in the *Journal of the American Medical Association,* argued that "medicine . . . has been the habitual critic of [the nurse's] development, and rightly so, because the physician is ultimately the only competent judge of the fitness of the nurse, and the chief sufferer . . . for her (sic) possible unfitness" (Beard, 1913, pp. 2149–2150).

In the 1960s when I worked as a hospital staff nurse, the doctor's idea of a "good nurse" was one who would precisely carry out his orders. Woe to the nurse who didn't. An angry doctor could march to the supervisor's office and demand that a nurse be fired. Physician wrath could be terrifying. On one occasion, still vivid in my memory, a doctor hurled a bedpan out the window of a patient's room. Doctors were permitted to have temper tantrums—throwing surgical instruments, yelling at nurses, orderlies, and other underlings—but such behavior was unthinkable for nurses. Nurses' anger was expressed only in interactions with each other, through indirect means such as nasty notes taped to locker doors or behind-the-scenes sabotage—the horizontal hostility we talked about earlier.

Nurses learned to "handle" doctors to avoid their ire by playing a devious "doctor-nurse game" described in an article by physician Leonard Stein (1967). The cardinal rule of the game was avoidance of open disagreement, and of course it was the nurse's job to make sure that disagreement did not erupt. As in a traditional marriage, in which the passive wife plants her idea so skillfully that her dominant husband believes he thought of it himself, so nurses were to communicate their recommendations to the doctor without appearing to make them. Making direct suggestions to a doctor would have been insolent and insulting. This "game" stifled nurses' intellect and creativity and probably had an adverse effect on patient care as well. The level and quality of physician-nurse interaction has been shown to affect patient outcomes (Knaus, Draper, Wagner, & Zimmerman, 1986).

In the 1970s, as the women's movement and the civil rights movement were shaking up entrenched power imbalances throughout the United States, some nurses became emboldened. In June 1975, a nurse at St. Agnes Hospital in Philadelphia refused to give a medication ordered by a doctor because she believed it to be harmful. The doctor-nurse confrontation that followed eventually led to the dismissal of the director of nursing. That part of the story wasn't unique. What followed the unfair firing of the director *was*. St. Agnes nurses protested for the director's reinstatement, and 30 courageous RNs resigned their jobs. Their story was picked up by the national media and was reported in *Modern Healthcare* (Cleary, 1975). The St. Agnes incident may have been the beginning of the end of the doctor-nurse game, because nurses weren't as willing to play anymore.

In the 1980s the AMA attempted to perpetuate its dominance at the bedside by creating a new group of hospital-trained workers—registered care technicians (RCTs)—whose primary responsibility would have been to carry out doctors' orders, presumably without giving them the flak that some better-educated "uppity" nurses were starting to do. But by this time nursing had enough political savvy and lobbying skill to defeat the RCT proposal.

Is the doctor-nurse game still being played? In some settings, yes. But when Stein, along with two physician coauthors, wrote a 1990 update, important changes had taken place. Physicians are no longer viewed as omnipotent. Medicine is less mystical and those who practice it are not held in awe. The gender composition in medicine is changing; physicians are increasingly likely to be female. Perhaps of greatest significance is the lessening education gap between physicians and nurses. In 1967, when Stein wrote his article, 90% of working nurses had been educated in hospital programs, such as the one I had attended. Less than 15% of nurses were being educated in such programs in 1990, and the majority of hospital staff nurses had received their education in community colleges or held baccalaureate degrees. When nursing education moved out of hospital-based schools to colleges and universities, students were no longer socialized to relate to doctors obsequiously. According to physician authors Stein, Watts, and Howell (1990), a few contemporary physicians still long wistfully for the return of the hierarchical doctor-nurse relationship, but "the forces of change are inexorable and universal" (p. 548). Stein et al. concluded their article by predicting a new, more equal, mutually interdependent relationship between physicians and nurses. They avowed that such a relationship would be beneficial to both disciplines: *"When a subordinate becomes liberated, there is the potential for the dominant one to become liberated too"* (p. 549).

The Continuing Turf Wars

While I am a strong advocate of developing mutually interdependent relationships with physicians, they are still our political adversaries on many occasions. It is ironic that perhaps the most collegial relationships nowadays are in the joint practices of physicians and nurse practitioners (NPs), yet physicians have consistently fought against NPs for years in nonproductive turf wars. They have fought against third-party reimbursement, prescription privileges, and independent functioning. Battles over changes in state laws are ongoing in some states. Not long ago in my state, legislation had been proposed to lift restrictions on nurse practitioners. The media campaign conducted by the Tennessee Medical Association (TMA) was downright nasty. On the cover of the TMA political action committee brochure was a large white duck with a stethoscope dangling from its neck. "Don't let reform duck up health care," read the brochure title. Inside the brochure, nonphysician care providers were discredited and referred to in derogatory terms such as "dubious birds" and "daffy ducks." The strong implication was that care provided by anyone other than a physician was "quackery." It was even suggested, in a "Legistat Fax" that TMA sent to its members, that the state board of nursing would not aggressively pursue violations by nurse practitioners. Through intense lobbying, the doctors successfully convinced legislators that the quality of patient care would suffer if nurses were allowed to practice independently, and the legislation was defeated.

Sexism reared its ugly head during the debate. How could female nurses be liberated from male physician control? One legislator made the following blatantly sexist comment: "It's hard not to like the ladies in white dresses with beautiful hats. But if you take the shackles off the nurse practitioners . . . you're taking a gamble." Use of the word *shackles* clearly brings images of slavery and bondage. I am happy to report, however, that the shackles eventually did come off. Furious over the physicians' demeaning, insulting propaganda, Tennessee nurses mounted a grassroots effort to revive and pass the bill. Newspapers across the state were inundated with letters from irate nurses. One year later, a standing-room-only crowd of nurses discovered what their collective anger could accomplish when they heard Representative Gary Odom proclaim: "Free at last, free at last, thank God Almighty, the nurse practitioners are free at last" (cited in Browning, 1994, p. 9).

But freedom is not all we want. As shown in our research data, nurses want to have satisfying relationships with our physician colleagues. Peggy Chinn (1991) explained:

We are seeking a quality in relationships that can exist only when we "count" as fully qualified, capable individuals. . . . What we are seeking is not so much freedom (although that certainly is an issue in many cases) as it is a *quality of connection* with everyone involved in our practice situation that endows us all with abilities to exercise our full human capacities—skill, judgment, and interaction (p. 254).

Looking to the Future

Interdisciplinary education for health professionals holds the greatest promise for creating egalitarian physician-nurse relationships. In a few academic health centers, medical and nursing students now take required courses together, in which they learn interviewing skills, history taking, physical assessment, epidemiology, community health, and wellness/illness concepts. Interdisciplinary electives such as ethics, adolescent health, and family violence are offered in some locales. Paired clinical assignments of medical and nursing students in rural clinics and other primary care settings have also been used (Larson, 1995). When physicians and nurses have studied together or seen patients side by side, hierarchy and territoriality are likely to diminish. These collaborative experiences promote collegiality and mutual respect. The Pew Health Professions Commission (1993) recommends widespread adoption of these innovations, but barriers such as scheduling, cost, and faculty attitudes remain. When Larson conducted a survey of 35 academic health centers in 1995, few had interdisciplinary courses available. In the meantime, while we wait for medical and nursing faculty to pursue additional collaborative initiatives, change is quietly occurring in practice settings. Work environments and roles are already changing as a result of managed care. Many doctors and nurses are working well together. Graduates of our NP programs at the University of Tennessee are eagerly sought by physicians to join their practices. In a recent speech, Lucille Joel, editor of the *American Journal of Nursing*, predicted that interdependent practice will be the reality of the future because the public will no longer tolerate turf battles among the professional groups.

Speaking of the public, let's turn our attention to our troubles in relating to patients.

6

Forging Alliances
With Patients

> There is no "simple" procedure or "minor" hospitaliza-
> tion. . . . The hospital bed reduces all to the lowest com-
> mon denominator. We have the privilege of connecting
> with people when they are most exposed and most de-
> fenseless. . . . With that privilege of intimacy comes the
> responsibility to make that connection a healing one.
>
> Sharon Adkins, MSN, RN

Much has been written about the emotional impact of illness, the vulnerability and powerlessness of patients, and their fears regarding pain,
mutilation, and mortality. But how often do we really stop to consider
what an invasion of privacy it is when we ask those "routine" questions
on admission to our facility? It is certainly not "routine" to the person
we are questioning to reveal his bowel habits, spiritual beliefs, substance
use, and sexual problems (even abuse) to a perfect stranger with a clip-
board. He is already being asked to bare his body and donate its blood
and urine, and we are trying to probe his psyche and soul as well. Every
blank on the assessment form must be filled. Nothing is sacred now.
And it won't be long until somebody else shows up and asks most of
those same questions again. Tubes, needles, and other devices of tor-
ture are soon to come.

It doesn't surprise me a bit, given the unpleasantness of so many in-
vasive things that we must do to patients, that negative images of
nurses abound. When nurses are female, as most still are, a plethora of
frightening and unpleasant images can be generated: old maids, battle-axes, and torturers (Muff, 1988). One particularly chilling image is

the formidable and controlling Nurse Ratched in *One Flew Over the Cuckoo's Nest,* who is more concerned with smooth functioning of the organization than the needs of patients (Kesey, 1973). Such an image crystallizes men's fear of powerful women, a fear acted out every day in situations involving male patients and female nurses. Rodgers (1982) points out that nursing, as a predominantly female occupation, conjures up the image of the nursing mother. The breast is the first object of human envy, and by extension, woman is therefore the first person envied. As a consequence, females in the nursing profession are "vulnerable to angry, envious, and destructive, although perhaps largely unconscious, impulses of the many others with whom we deal—patients, as well as physicians and other colleagues" (Rodgers, 1982, p. 347).

Female nurses also evoke sexual fantasies in male patients. Nursing, by its very nature of having to care for patients' bodily needs, violates normal social rules regarding bodily contact. Furthermore, there may be exaggerated expectations based on nurses' warm and caring attitude (Robbins, Bender, & Finnis, 1997). Judging by greeting cards, the stereotypical image of a sexy nurse is a woman with a minuscule brain, luscious lips, and generous breasts. Patients do act on their fantasies by making sexual remarks or touching nurses inappropriately—even if we don't look much like the caricatures of nurses on the greeting cards. Who among us hasn't been asked if we would like to get in a patient's bed? New research (Libbus & Bowman, 1997) shows that such behavior remains common, despite widespread societal consciousness-raising about sexual harassment in the last few years.

The public's most common stereotype or image of a male nurse is that he must be gay (Williams, 1995). While there are gay men in the profession, it is ludicrous for patients to make an assumption about sexual orientation solely on the basis of nontraditional career choice. But the common reasoning is that if a man engages in nurturing human service work, he is effeminate—a "sure sign" of homosexuality. Male nurses experience the gamut of harassment, from outright propositions and cruel taunting to covert snickers and chortles as they go down the hall. To "display" heterosexuality, some male nurses wear wedding bands or deliberately mention their wives and children while giving patient care.

In contrast to these images of nurses as battle-axes, sexpots, or sexual deviants, there are equally erroneous idealized ones enshrined in the human psyche: nurse as angel of mercy, handmaiden to the physician, pure and virginal woman in white (Muff, 1982). The strongest of these is probably the saintly Nightingale image of the lady with the lamp, weary but driven by her enormous compassion to continue her rounds far into the night. (We nurses have internalized this one too, driving ourselves like the indefatigable Nightingale to work one more shift, see one more patient, give one more heaping tablespoonful of TLC.)

Not surprisingly, given the irrational expectations that these various images generate in patients, we nurses often fail to do what is expected of us. Angels and saints we are not. Furthermore, discontent among consumers is increasing as health care organizations place pressure on their scaled-down nursing staffs to increase productivity through "speed-ups" (see Chapter 1). Fifty-five percent of nurses in a 1996 *American Journal of Nursing* survey reported an increase in patient and family complaints over the past year (Shindul-Rothschild, Berry, & Long-Middleton, 1996). What is it like for you when your patient becomes angry at you?

WHEN THE PATIENT IS ANGRY AT YOU

Once I was in a patient's room helping another nurse. I do not recall exactly what was said, but the patient became upset and angry. The other nurse told the patient, "I'll go get you something for your nerves." Turning to me, she said, "Will you see if the social worker can come up and talk with her?" I was stunned. Why did we need the Ativan or the social worker?

As shown in this student's report of an anger incident, nurses can find angry patients quite threatening, and common responses are medicating them or trying to get someone else to handle them. Nurse behaviors of disconnecting (Smith & Hart, 1994) and becoming frustrated and angry in return (Podrasky & Sexton, 1988) are documented in the research literature. Smith and Hart's grounded theory study of med-surg nurses sheds light on the process of managing angry patient situations. Disconnecting from the patient occurred when nurses appraised the anger as a personal attack ("She would call us names . . . call us 'whores' and other very bad names and I felt very degraded"). Nurses did not understand the patient's reality and reacted with shock and a sense of being off balance ("It took me totally off guard"). As they struggled to understand, they felt self-blame ("Maybe it was something I overlooked"). Some of the nurses believed that dealing with angry patients was beyond their expertise ("Except for psych nurses, nobody knows and nobody feels able to cope"). As their own anger arose, they feared its power and sought to hide it. If it escaped, they felt ashamed. After all, they had learned that "good nurses" do not get angry at their patients. Nurses tried strategies such as taking a timeout, transferring blame, seeking peer support, and "returning to smooth," which meant repairing the relationship with the patient. The smoothing did not involve talking about the anger incident, but rather acting as though nothing had happened—which I view as a less-than-ideal resolution of the angry episode.

Not all nurses disconnected from angry patients. Three of the study participants were able to remain with the patient, exploring the anger, analyzing its cause, and trying not to take it personally. Smith and Hart attributed this ability to remain connected during anger to the amount of experience these nurses had (experience of the study participants ranged widely, from 1 to 21 years). Therefore, they concluded their article on a hopeful note that more effective responses to patient anger could be developed by nurses over time. That conclusion certainly fits with my view.

Sometimes specific patients will present you with an opportunity to learn. Much of what I know about establishing trust with paranoid patients I learned while working with Evelyn and Gladys. I learned about delusions from David and Toby, borderlines from Maureen, and suicide from a woman named Hope who no longer had any hope. Stephanie Hart, a Minnesota staff nurse, learned about angry patients from Liz:

> *Initially, she was a difficult patient, her anger and aggressiveness delivered with a swift, biting tongue. . . . She never uttered a "please" or a "thank you." . . . Why, I wondered, did she refuse important procedures; why wouldn't she conform to my therapeutic regimen? . . . She angrily rejected my efforts, yet expected me to return to her room on demand. . . . Our relationship slowly evolved with each isolated moment of intimacy, each small revelation about her family life, childhood experiences, and dreams. . . . Only when she was gone did I fully realize what she had come to mean to me. . . . While I thought I was doing all the giving, Liz was giving something back to me: a lesson I didn't learn in nursing school and couldn't gain even from the most comprehensive inservice or the wisest of mentors. In the end, she taught me to recognize the helplessness and fear behind a patient's anger and anxiety and to realize that rejection may be a manifestation of the inability to cope. (Hart, 1997, p. 54)*

Read on for some strategies that may be helpful to you in defusing patient anger.

WHAT TO DO WHEN THE PATIENT IS ANGRY

1. Help the patient to discover why he or she is angry. Anger is always aroused for a reason. Anxiety and frustration are common when individuals must undergo scary and uncomfortable procedures and put up with depersonalizing institutional routines. Direct your attention to the patient's sense of threat or fear, speaking in a calm and reassuring tone. Listen to the patient express his or her feelings and acknowledge their legitimacy. Don't interrupt the patient as he or she articulates these grievances. Tell the patient you understand what he or she is saying (to make sure, paraphrase what you heard and ask if you are on target). Help the patient articulate what he or she needs or wants to become comfortable. Work with the patient to develop a mutually satisfactory plan to get these needs met.

2. When people complain, don't explain. Patients do not want an explanation, even if it is a very good one. They just want their needs met. A typical scenario might involve a hospitalized patient who has been waiting a long time for an injection for pain. So he growls into the intercom: "Where the hell is my shot?" Your worst response goes something like this: "There's no need to be hateful. We are really short of help this evening. There are five people ahead of you and you'll just have to wait." This response labels the patient (hateful), explains (short of help), and creates added anxiety (with five people ahead of him, God knows when his shot will finally come). You have compounded the misery of an individual who is hurting and angry.

   So what's a better approach? Validate the complaint: "I can see why you are upset." Apologize, then focus on what can be done rather than what hasn't been done. If possible, assure the patient that you will take care of the complaint yourself. He's still not going to be a happy camper if you tell him, "I'll try to find your nurse," because a hurting patient already imagines that his nurse has departed for Outer Mongolia. Besides, the delay in receiving the analgesic already seems interminable. I suggest that you say, "I'm really sorry that you've had to wait. I will take care of it right now."

3. When the patient is really angry at someone else—and you are just the convenient target at whom it is directed—teach the patient how to communicate his or her concerns to the real target. This is basically a matter of teaching assertive communication. For example, your patient's pain is unrelieved by the analgesic ordered by

her doctor. Help the patient to speak up for herself: "Ms. Jones, I think it is very important that you tell the doctor that your new pain medication is not relieving you. Tell him exactly where your pain is and how it feels. He should be coming to the unit to make rounds shortly. I'll make sure he comes to see you first." As patients develop confidence that they can effectively communicate and influence their plan of care, they are less likely to feel helpless and angry.

4. Be alert to transference phenomena. Is a certain patient reacting to you the way he reacted to his critical mother or punitive father? Talk with him about important figures in his life and previous experiences with caregivers. The patient may have no conscious awareness that he is transferring strong emotion about a childhood figure to you. As he gets to know you better, and you steadfastly meet his needs for care, he will be able to see you as a unique individual and behave less angrily.

5. When you must set limits on a patient's behavior, there are ways to do it without provoking anger and aggression. The worst way to set limits, according to a study by Lancee, Gallop, McCay, and Toner (1995) is making a statement that belittles the patient ("You act like a child, you get treated like a child"). This type of statement by the nurse almost always generates considerable anger. In contrast, affective involvement, or establishing rapport and relationship, is correlated with the least amount of patient anger. Offering a patient options is also an effective strategy. Avoid preachy platitudes like "We practice the golden rule here: Treat others as you want to be treated."

6. If you are at your wit's end dealing with an angry, demanding, patient, use the consultants available in your facility, such as a psychiatric liaison nurse, social worker, psychologist, or chaplain. If possible, schedule a team conference to discuss the patient and problem-solve. There are many options to consider: rotating the nurses assigned to the patient so that no one becomes completely drained, recruiting volunteers to spend time with him, perhaps moving him to a semiprivate room. Make sure everyone on the team is informed of the new approach so that staff behavior toward the patient is consistent.

7. Never lose sight of the potential for an angry patient to become violent. Be alert for clenched fists, pacing, and other signs that a patient may become assaultive. Violence is more apt to occur when a patient is under the influence of drugs or alcohol or has impaired ability to think clearly and behave rationally because of organic

brain disease, psychosis, brain trauma, mental retardation, or other disorders affecting the central nervous system. Paranoid individuals may attack you in what they perceive as self-defense against an incipient attack by you. Your goal in dealing with potentially violent patients is safety—of the patient, staff, and yourself. Keep a safe distance from the patient. Don't ever let an agitated, angry patient stand between you and the door. Speak to the patient in a calm, reassuring way. Make sure someone else on the staff knows where you are and is ready to come to your aid if needed. However, in my experience, it can be very frightening to a patient if you panic and call security prematurely. In several situations on our psych unit, just as I was making progress subduing an agitated patient, a technician erred by calling security. When the big, burly security guards came tromping into the room, the patient completely lost control. I believe that the use of force or restraints should be a last resort. Every health care facility should have a plan for dealing with violent behavior that can be mobilized in a crisis situation. This has become increasingly important as violence has escalated in our society.

WHAT TO DO WHEN YOU ARE ANGRY AT THE PATIENT

In the workshops that I've conducted, I've heard vivid examples of nurses' anger at patients, particularly those who were not "good." As we discussed in Chapter 3, "good" patients are not demanding and are properly grateful for our ministrations. Our beliefs and values about other aspects of patient behavior fuel anger too. Listen to Bonnie Hartman, a public health nurse:

> *I get angry at some of the clients we see, particularly those who are demanding, complain about having to wait, and those who don't even take a bath before they come. They miss appointments or are late because they overslept. Then they demand to be seen when they come. And they don't even have a job—they just overslept. I'd like to oversleep or come and go as I please. But I'm here working as hard as I can to get the clients seen so they won't complain about the long wait or miss their soap opera!*

There is a tone of moral indignation in this nurse's account of her anger at patients. Notice that Bonnie thinks that the patients should bathe before they come to the health department. Several nurse authors, including Myra Levine, have written about nurses' views regarding cleanliness: " 'Unclean' has long meant more than merely dirty. But it was the Victorians who married cleanliness to godliness, and with it a moral halo that hovers over many of the decisions individuals make for themselves. . . . The poor are castigated if they appear dirty because, as the argument goes, soap is cheap" (Levine, 1970, p. 2108). I'm sure you have heard nurses say things like, "The least these people can do is keep clean."

While personal hygiene is undoubtedly important, what some nurses mean by "clean" is a particular kind of shiny, well-scrubbed, shaved, and deodorized ideal that only a tiny minority of the citizens of the world can achieve. Foreign visitors to our home are often astonished that we wasteful Americans take showers every single day—sometimes more than one per day—and wash our clothes after every single wearing. There is no such stringent standard in their cultures, nor is there sufficient water. And we don't have to go abroad to gain a different perspective. My own views about cleanliness have been badly shaken on more than one occasion when my nursing assignment took me into a patient's home that had no running water, or into a housing project where laundered clothes could not be hung out on the line to dry because the clothespins would immediately be stolen. I wondered how often I would do a big laundry if I had to wash the clothes in the bathtub and hang them on the backs of the chairs to dry.

Bonnie also decries the indolence of her patients who "don't even have a job," unlike Bonnie, who arises early and works hard to serve them. She clearly espouses the Protestant work ethic and makes a judgment that someone who is not working is less virtuous. While we can surely empathize with her sense of unfairness (why must her freedom be constrained when the patients can come and go as they please?), a note of caution must be sounded. It is easy for care providers of one culture or social class to assume that their own values, norms, and practices are superior to those of other groups. Because the nursing profession in the United States historically has drawn its recruits largely from the white Euro-American middle class, the cultural values of this segment of the population have permeated nursing philosophy, textbooks, and clinical practices. Our way of thinking and doing things seems "normal" and "right," and we make judgments about people who do not conform to our views. We understand neither the idleness of the rich, who fly from one seasonal pleasure spot to another to ski, sail, and sunbathe, nor the idleness of the poor, who "blithely" accept checks from the government and other kinds of assistance from social welfare agencies. We wonder why the poor can't pull themselves up by their bootstraps. Isn't this the land of equal opportunity?

Consider the following white Euro-American middle-class values that have been well entrenched: (1) achievement, occupational and financial success, status consciousness; (2) speed, activity, efficiency; (3) youth, beauty, health, self-reliance; (4) science and the use of technology; (5) materialism, consumerism, use of disposable items; (6) conformity to the group simultaneously with rugged individualism; (7) social and geographical mobility; and (8) competitive and aggressive behavior instead of cooperation (Murray & Zentner, 1979). However, many of these ethnocentric values are being questioned now. Individuals of diverse racial, ethnic, and cultural groups are becoming increasingly visible and influential in politics, business, and health care.

Returning to our discussion of patient characteristics that provoke nurses' wrath, noncompliance with the treatment regimen is another anger trigger. When we interviewed female nurses (Smith et al., 1996), anger was particularly leveled at patients who were self-destructive:

> *Addicts, suicidal patients—I could not help but feel a certain amount of anger. You've charcoaled them out because they've overdosed for the third time in a row—OK, fine, do the job next time. Don't call 911 . . . taking up tax dollars and nurse time, it's a waste of resources.*

> *You have whiners and complainers that are taking up your time because they're on the buzzer all the time. . . . Whiners of any kind anger me . . . malingerers . . . "oh my head hurts, this hurts, that hurts, my big toe, oh please scratch it; you know." Those [patients] anger me because they're taking my time away and I only have a certain allotment for a certain amount of patients.*

One proposed explanation for nurses' anger toward patients is that "women nurses who have been dominated by others and operate from a male-normed perspective may exact revenge for their own powerlessness in the relationships formed with clients" (Caroline & Bernhard, 1994, p. 85). However, this explanation fails to account for similar behavior we observed when we studied male nurses (Brooks et al., 1996). Here are some examples from our male nurse data. Mike Evans was angry at noncompliant patients who refused to change their behaviors (smoking, diet, etc.), resulting in repeated admissions to his unit:

They come in near death and you nurse them back. . . . Two months down the road you see them again in the same shape. . . . If they're not a moron, they can listen to instructions and dose their insulin or follow a diet, but they continue all the things that bring them in in horrible shape. . . . And I have to take care of them. It's disgusting. I wanted to say, "If you're not going to follow any of our advice or do anything to help yourself, then why don't you just stay home and die?"

On one occasion, Mike said he walked out, unable to take care of a patient:

The patient had chronic obstructive pulmonary disease and then developed laryngeal cancer, had a laryngectomy, had a tracheostomy, and was still smoking. He would smoke through his tracheostomy. The first time I walked in and saw him smoking, I just had to walk out in disgust. I couldn't take care of him.

Tom Parker is angered by demanding patients who want more from their nurse than he is able to give. He spoke of a "CD" (chemically dependent patient) who was making rapid-fire demands:

This person's demeanor, his whole personality just rubbed me the wrong way. The patient had a whining type of attitude, but very persistent, the kind of thing that just pecks and pecks and pecks at you, without a letup. It was the demandingness that really bothered me; it was just rapid fire, demanding attention almost in a hysterical way. He was asking for something that I could not deliver.

Ron Murray described an anger episode with a patient who had been in restraints. After telling the patient that he would undo the restraints "as long as you are good," he caught her out of bed:

She was up walking around the room with the IV cord stretched just as far as it would stretch. And she's real hard to stick. . . . It was aggravating, plus the stress of all the other patients that you've got . . . and here you've got one that's acting out. . . . I really think she knew what she was doing.

Nurses' anger at patients who are not "good" can be quite virulent, as shown in this final example, taken from Larson (1987). The nurse in this situation described herself as "burned out," which I take to mean that she was at the limit of her patience and tolerance. Her overreaction to a balky baby who "wouldn't eat" scared her and left her feeling guilty:

> *A couple of weeks ago, I was feeling really burned out and I had a newborn who wouldn't eat, and when I gavaged him, he spit all the formula back up, and I gritted my teeth and became so angry at the baby. It really scared me because I felt like I could have hit him or something for not eating. I waited about 15 minutes and then tried to feed him again, feeling much better, but I really felt guilty for a long time" (Larson, 1987, p. 23).*

The anger at patients in these examples is antithetical to a therapeutic nurse- patient relationship. Many of these nurses, in fact, have rejected their noncompliant patients and no longer wish to remain in relationship with them because the patients "won't try to help themselves." I argue that even when patients refuse to follow our directives, it is unethical to abandon them. When I teach students, I often share with them an article that I have found especially useful. The article, which appeared in the *New England Journal of Medicine,* identified four types of difficult patients and gave suggestions for dealing with them (Groves, 1978). Let me say, before we go on, that I do not especially like the labels the author gave these patients, but I think all of us will recognize the behaviors described. Here are the four types of difficult patients and recommended strategies.

1. *Dependent clingers.* These are patients who appear to have bottomless needs. In the inpatient setting, they are the ones referred to as "on the buzzer all the time." They may flatter caregivers by saying things like "You're so good to me. What would I do without you?" Eventually they evoke aversion in their caregivers because their requests escalate from mild ones to repeated cries for affection, explanation, and/or analgesics. As the nurse, you should set limits, give the patient regular appointments at specific intervals (or specify reasonable intervals when you will return to give care, if you are in an inpatient setting), and remind the patient not to call at other times unless it is an emergency. When reassured of regular, consistent attention, these patients will not need to keep escalating their cries for help.

2. *Entitled demanders.* These individuals use intimidation and guilt induction to obtain care. They may threaten their care providers with litigation. They are unaware of their deep dependency needs and fear of abandonment. The entitlement is an attempt to preserve

the integrity of the self during terrifying illness. The nurse's approach should be to support the entitlement because that reassures the patient: "You are entitled to the very best care, and you will get it." Hostile responses will only add to the patient's terror of abandonment.

3. *Manipulative help-rejecters.* These patients feel that no interventions will help them, and they often report back to you (smugly) that the treatments didn't work. If one symptom is alleviated, they will develop another, because they want to keep the relationship with the caregiver. These individuals evoke feelings of inadequacy and guilt in caregivers. The suggested approach? Share their pessimism. In a low-key way, tell them you're not sure this treatment will work. Don't appear invested in the treatment ("Let's give this a try"). Tell the patient that regular checkups will be necessary (allays fear of abandonment), and be consistent and firm.

4. *Self-destructive deniers.* These are among the most difficult patients of all, because they are either consciously suicidal or unconsciously self-murderous through behaviors such as heavy drinking despite esophageal varices and hepatic failure. Caregivers may wish that the person would die and get it over with. These individuals are profoundly dependent but have given up hope of ever having their needs met. They seem to glory in their own destruction and enjoy defeating attempts to preserve their lives. The recommended approach is to fight your impulse to abandon the such a patient, and after ruling out if a treatable depression exists, then consider the patient as you would any other terminal patient. Continue to preserve life and maintain the nurse-patient relationship as long as possible.

What is important with all four types of patients is not how you feel but how you behave. It is understandable that you may have negative feelings. Acknowledge these feelings and harmlessly discharge them, but continue to give compassionate care to the patient. Remaining in relationship with a difficult or self-destructive patient can be a tremendous learning experience of oneself. I recall Hildegard Peplau pointing out that nursing is always a learning experience of oneself as well as of the other individual involved in the interaction. Patients often evoke emotions and memories that their caregivers would rather avoid. But when we shut out a patient because of this, we are closing off access to an important part of ourselves (Stein, cited in L. Dossey, 1984). When a patient evokes strong emotion in you, it should always be a cue to (1) look closely at the defensive maneuvers the patient may be using and (2) carefully analyze your own strong reaction. Is it your own helplessness to control the patient that generates your anger? Is it your own fear and denial of death that makes it so difficult to be with someone who is longing for it?

In an atmosphere of collegial trust and support, you can ventilate excess anger and frustration to other nurses in the setting. I found this a necessity in a psychiatric inpatient unit, especially when working with patients who were manipulative and intent on testing limits, splitting staff, and generally creating turmoil. I was fortunate to work for a number of years with a very special group of people who talked freely in staff meetings about their own issues with difficult patients. Together, we found ways to maintain a therapeutic milieu—and our own sanity.

WHY WE NEED TO MANAGE OUR ANGER AT PATIENTS

There is no question that sometimes our anger at patients is justifiable. But it is important to manage our anger at patients, even intransigent and obnoxious ones, more effectively. The first, and foremost, reason is to preserve the therapeutic relationship, without which nothing else of any consequence can be accomplished. As Myra Levine (1970) put it, "Whether [the patient's] difficulties are truly self-inflicted or quite beyond his control, no patient is served by moralistic judgments. Nursing care laced with censure is not nursing and not caring. . . . Nursing intervention can provide a transcendent way to a more inclusive humanity for the patient and the nurse. All patients deserve that effort" (pp. 2018, 2111). The second reason why we need to get a handle on our anger is that it is impossible to estimate the ripple effect in that patient's life from one interaction with a nurse. Jean Watson (1988) talked about the potential ramifications when nurse and patient come together:

> *Two persons (nurse and other) together with their unique life histories and phenomenal fields in a human care transaction comprise an event. An event, such as an actual occasion of human care, is a focal point in space and time from which experience and perception are taking place, but the actual occasion of caring has a field of its own that is greater than the occasion itself. As such, the process can go beyond itself, yet arise from aspects of itself that become part of the life history of each person, as well as part of some larger, deeper, complex pattern of life. (p. 58)*

I know that you have experienced "the process going beyond," as I have, when you run across a former patient who thanks you for something you did that had a profound and lasting influence. You might not have thought much about what seemed a very simple intervention at the time. One day a woman came up to me and said, "I still remember what you taught me about anxiety. I carry that little card with the stages of anxiety in my wallet to this day. I used to think I just had "bad nerves" like everybody in my family. But you showed me that I can do something when I'm getting too nervous. I stop what I'm doing and start my breathing exercise." I honestly didn't recognize the patient or recall that I had written a card for her about the stages of anxiety, but she remembered me. People do remember their nurses, because so often nurses are in their lives during agonizing times of crisis or epiphanies that remain vivid in memory. People also generalize beyond their experience with one nurse to the profession as a whole.

In each and every patient encounter, there is the potential for your patient (and his or her significant others) to form a lasting impression of nursing. Think of a restaurant where you got bad service from a surly or indifferent server. Did you go back? Probably not, even if you know that you should not judge the place or its servers on the basis of one experience. So too a patient who waits a long time for an injection for pain, then gets it in a perfunctory, mechanistic manner, is going to remember that and form judgments about "nurses who are only in it for the paycheck and don't really care." If you ask patients, they can tell you stories of incidents decades ago when a nurse was unkind to them.

Or perhaps the nurse was not unkind, just mechanical, doing the tasks with no recognition of the patient's individuality. During hospitalization for surgery, I remember how it felt when a nurse came into the room and looked at my IV, then turned and left without ever looking at me. Sidney Jourard (1971) called the bedside manner displayed by many nurses "a peculiar kind of inauthentic behavior. . . . Some nurses always smile, others hum, and still others answer all patients' questions about medications with the automatic phrase, 'This will make you feel better'" (pp. 179–180). Jourard dryly commented that the performance sometimes functions as an emetic. He understood why nurses may armor themselves to maintain professional detachment: "If the 'armor' is effective, it permits the nurse to go about her duties unaffected by any disturbing feelings of pity, anger, inadequacy, or insecurity" (p. 181). The problem, of course, is that the nurse's impersonal bedside manner, whether slightly chilly or falsely jolly, obliterates the individuality of patients. They feel dehumanized, like Matt Stolick did, when the nurse made a canned statement while preparing him for surgery:

"It sure is cold in this room," I thought to myself as I awaited my upcoming knee surgery. I was naked under a flimsy robe, nervous, and just wanted to get the whole thing over with. A pre-op nurse strutted into the room. At my quiet demeanor and nonverbal avoidance of her initial greeting she offered, "Don't worry; we'll try to keep the pain to a minimum." I was appalled at this statement. I didn't say anything for fear of overreacting. And yet I felt violated in so many ways. This nurse was incredibly presumptuous, and her way of treating me from this first exchange was alienating and depersonalizing.

What do patients really want? Like the old song, little things mean a lot. Matt shared with me a second story, from the same hospitalization, that illustrates the importance of little things:

The nurse who was assigned to me came in during dinnertime, greeted me with a smile, and asked if there was anything she could get me. There was a Coke on the tray, and I told her that I would really like a Pepsi instead. She laughed and apologized, saying that they only had Coke. . . . Early in the morning I was sitting up in bed, waiting to see my physician. My nurse came in with her jacket on, ready to leave for home. She had a smile on her face and a Pepsi in her hand. She told me that she had gotten it downstairs and wanted to give it to me before she left. After that I was much more comfortable in the hospital, in light of this compassionate gesture on the nurse's part.

Matt's story about the Pepsi reminds me of the innumerable small acts of kindness Nightingale performed for the soldiers at Scutari. She found time to make nightly rounds in all the wards, stayed with the men during amputations, wrote letters to their families in England, and set up a recreation room for convalescents. The men adored her. I have often wondered what sustained Nightingale at Scutari during the discouraging early days of filthy conditions, woefully inadequate supplies, and opposition from army medical officers. I believe she found her sustenance in the one-to-one interactions she had with the soldiers themselves (Thomas, 1993a). In Nightingale's later years, when she was an elderly invalid, what she remembered most about the horror of Scutari was the soldiers who were her patients. She was still corresponding with the survivors of the Balaclava Charge in 1900, more than 40 years after the Crimean War had ended. Her lifework was epitomized in these words from a note she once wrote: *"I stand at the altar of the murdered men, and, while I live, I fight their cause."*

FORGING ALLIANCES WITH PATIENTS

The public demanded nursing after the acclaim of Nightingale's patients at Scutari—the whole world wanted those wonderful Nightingale nurses. Requests poured in for graduates of the Nightingale Training School to come and start nursing education programs in other countries. It is this kind of public demand that may be our saving grace in today's battle to preserve and strengthen professional nursing. I believe that forging alliances with patients should be one of the most crucial elements in our strategic plan. Heaven knows, consumers are just about fed up with the other players scrambling for their business in today's health care arena. In 1997 the National Coalition on Health Care released a national survey of Americans' perceptions regarding the health care system. The survey's findings clearly indicate a crisis of consumer confidence:

- Seventy-nine percent of respondents agree that "there is something seriously wrong with our health care system."
- More than half (57%) believed that "hospital care is not very good."
- Less than half (44%) said they had "confidence in the health care system to take care of me."
- Eight in ten believed that "quality medical care has become unaffordable for the average American," that "hospitals have cut corners to save money," that "quality care is often compromised by insurance companies to save money," and that "quality of medical care has gone down while costs have increased" ("Survey Finds Consumer Confidence . . . ," 1997, p. 5).

Other recent surveys show that two out of three Americans no longer hold physicians in high regard and see health care facilities as slightly better than automotive repair shops, but less satisfactory than supermarkets and airlines (Aiken, 1992). However, despite the potential for angry conflicts between patients and their nurses that we have been examining, studies show that nursing still enjoys highly positive regard from the public (Hart, 1990). In fact, most people say they would like to receive more health care from nurses. Additionally, the public is concerned about the increased use of unlicensed health workers. Eighty-five percent of participants in a 1996 national survey felt that it was inappropriate for unlicensed personnel to draw blood and insert catheters, IVs, and other tubes, and 74% said these workers should not give medications (American Nurses Association, 1996). Through the years, I have been struck by how interested people are in the work that we do. Casual social conversations often elicit remarks such as, "Your job must be fascinating" or "I wish I could have been a nurse." Books such as *Just a Nurse* (Kraegel & Kachoyeanos, 1989) capture the interest of laypersons as well as nurse readers and provide a glimpse of the everyday heroism in nursing practice.

The public has responded positively to recent media campaigns, such as the ANA's national "Every Patient Deserves a Nurse" initiative and the Massachusetts Statewide Campaign for Safe Care. In 1994 the quality of nursing care in Massachusetts was viewed as rapidly deteriorating. The number of RNs had decreased dramatically (and the number of UAPs had increased) in institutions that were "reengineering" and "restructuring." In September of that year, members of the Massachusetts Nurses Association (MNA) unanimously agreed to begin a formal campaign to educate consumers about what was happening. Hundreds of RNs from around the state participated in media training so that they would be prepared to communicate effectively to the public. When the ANA held its huge Nurses' March on Washington in the spring of 1995, Massachusetts nurses joined in and alerted radio and television stations back home to cover the event. The MNA sent notices to RNs in hospitals and long-term care facilities, inviting them to call in to talk shows to share their own concerns about patient care quality. They did. Since then, Massachusetts nurses have staged rallies at the state house, written letters to newspapers, given information to citizens during blood pressure screenings at malls, and developed a legislative package of five bills. This story has a happy ending: The public—and the legislature—got the message, and the first bill in that legislative package passed on December 30, 1996. The ABC network's "Nightline" focused an entire segment on the replacement of RNs with UAPs, featuring the MNA president (Schildmeier, 1997).

Just as the Massachusetts nurses have come forward with their stories, so too have consumers and their families coming forward to support us. Jack Strunk, whose wife died after a routine hysterectomy (see Chapter 1), has become a staunch ally of the nursing profession because of this tragedy. You will recall that Rebecca Strunk had developed a massive infection as a result of a nicked bowel during the surgery, but she did not have RNs caring for her, and the unlicensed aides hired to take their places did not recognize the infection symptoms. Mr. Strunk has become a crusader against cuts in RN staffs to save costs. When the American Nurses Association held a recent press conference at the National Press Club, Jack Strunk was there to share his story. In a moving statement,

Strunk, fighting back tears, said, "I am here to represent my wife who can't be here because the hospital put the dollar ahead of her care" (Canavan, 1997a, p. 12).

SHALL WE ADOPT A NEW SLOGAN?

As we continue to develop alliances with patients, Kitson (1997) suggests that we adopt a new slogan: "We'll be there for you." She believes that this slogan conveys an image of nurse-as-companion that will be appealing to the public. The idea of nurse-as-companion is taken from the work of Campbell (1984), who characterized the nurse's role as "skilled companion," bringing together the technical skills or "doing to" and the caring presence or "being with." I am not sure the slogan "We'll be there for you" communicates this whole concept, or whether Campbell's concept of nursing actually has sufficient depth. Somehow it sounds shallow compared to Martin Buber's I-thou relationship or Sidney Jourard's view that nursing is a special case of loving. A recent qualitative study, involving 10 psychiatric RNs, revealed that the nurses felt a deep, enriching connection with their patients, going beyond the "patientness" of the person. The relationship was transformative for the patients, opening up new possibilities for them and empowering them (Pieranunzi, 1997). I'm not sure any slogan or media sound bite could capture what this kind of nurse-patient relationship means to those human beings who are suffering. Such a relationship increases a patient's sense of being worthy of caring and promotes his or her recovery from illness. Perhaps consumers who have been the recipients of magnificent nursing care just need to share their stories with loved ones, legislators, and CEOs of health care organizations. To this day, the power of narrative has never been surpassed for its ability to engage attention and emotion: You will probably remember Matt's stories long after you have forgotten the rest of the material in this chapter. Nursing's "closeness to the customer of health care," as Donna Shalala has put it, is our greatest asset. Nurses must be vocal in policy debates to ensure that all customers continue to have access to professional nursing care.

Nurses have one foot high in the tower of knowledge, one in the dust and grit of human need. This closeness to the customer of health care is not only a distinctive value and philosophy of nursing, but a strength that can be used to create a vision for health care organizations.

III

Healing
Ourselves

7

Examining What We Learned About Anger While Growing Up

> Our task, then, is to strengthen our consciousness
> of ourselves, to find centers of strength within
> ourselves which will enable us to stand despite
> the confusion and bewilderment around us.
>
> Rollo May

Having devoted attention in the last section of the book to connecting with others, we move into important material on self-healing in the next three chapters. Rollo May has outlined our task quite well. But before examining new ways of thinking, feeling, and behaving that strengthen us and promote healing, it's necessary to reflect on how we got the way we are. Before we were ever nurses, we were learning emotional habits along gendered lines. Levinson (1996) proposed a concept called "gender splitting" that I find more useful than "gender differences," because it more accurately depicts the splitting asunder or rigid division between masculine and feminine in human life. Gender splitting has been pervasive, occurring in virtually every society in the history of the human species. What is sanctioned for masculine and feminine gender roles varies according to historical period, social class, and other factors, but there is always gender splitting. The splitting operates in institutions, family life, and the individual human psyche.

Growing boys and girls are rapidly inculcated with societal norms about men's work and women's work, men's strength and women's weakness, and other stereotypical polarities. So too they learn the gendered rules of emotional expression. Lots of forces conspire to produce the traditional "insensitive male" and "overly emotional female." While emotional habits are modified by later experiences, early childhood learning instills much of what is considered "normal" for masculine and feminine gender roles. What did you learn about anger while growing up? Think about your own experiences as I review some of the literature.

IT STARTS WITH PINK AND BLUE
RECEIVING BLANKETS

From infancy on, parents apply different contingencies to the behaviors of sons and daughters, showing more acceptance of anger expression by sons (Birnbaum & Croll, 1984). Research shows that mothers emphasize anger more frequently when making up stories for their preschool sons than for their daughters (Greif, Alvarez, & Ulman, 1981). Boys are actually stimulated to aggressive action by their fathers from ages as young as 11/2 to 2 years (Miller, 1983), although the expression of other emotions, such as fear and sadness, is discouraged. Fathers, by instruction and example, get the message across to their sons that they must not ever be cowardly or weak. By the age of 3, boys wrestle, kick, push, shove, and hit far more than girls do (Fagot, Leinbach, & Hagan, 1986). Even throwing or breaking things may be condoned, because "boys will be boys."

In contrast, girls are allowed to be more emotional, as long as they are unaggressive (Block, 1973). With daughters, mothers emphasize that aggressive behavior may hurt people. A girl may be told, "If you can't say anything nice, just don't say anything at all." The child watches her mother playing the part of family peacemaker, skillfully placating her father to maintain a harmonious household. She is learning what Jessie Bernard (1981) called the ethos of "women's world" with its prescription that females help, agree, comply, understand, and passively accept. Expressing anger is not consistent with this ethos. What is the result of this early inculcation of cultural rules for gendered emotional behavior? By preschool age, happiness, sadness, fear, and general emotionality are more evident in girls, while anger and aggression are more characteristic of boys (Brody, 1985).

Television shows, movies, and other powerful socializing influences outside the family take up where parents leave off. Male TV characters express significantly more anger than female characters (Birnbaum &

Croll, 1984). History lessons in school portray aggressive men as heroes, while aggressive women are evil queens or wicked witches. Stories that form the foundation of our Western Judeo-Christian tradition identify women as the source of all evil. From Eve, who bit the apple, to Pandora, who foolishly opened the box, these stories teach that when women assert themselves, harm results (Wolf, 1993). The contrast between the stories of Eve and Prometheus is notable. When Prometheus defied Zeus and stole fire for human use, he was declared a hero. But when Eve defied God, she was condemned as evil and evicted from the Garden of Eden (Polster, 1992).

Boys and girls learn many lessons while playing. Competitive games and other rough-and-tumble experiences on the playground teach boys that life is a contest in which they need to stay one up. Meanwhile, girls, through cooperative activities with other girls who are good friends, learn that community is important (Tannen, 1990). When boys and girls play with one another, boys establish dominance early—as early as 33 months. Psychologists Carol Jacklin and Eleanor Maccoby (1978) studied the interaction between pairs of 33-month-olds. Whenever the boys were paired with girls, they clearly dominated play, grabbing, pushing, and ignoring the girls' protests. In fact, the boys were so unresponsive to the girls' protests that the girls usually just gave up, standing on the sidelines and letting the boys monopolize the toys. Sociologist Barrie Thorne (1993) watched an older group of school-age children at play, documenting boys' continued domination and girls' subservience. Boys controlled more space, more often violated girls' activities, and treated girls as "contaminating." Over time, girls learned to tighten and tense their bodies so they will take up less space, to tolerate interruptions of their speech and their activities, to hesitate, apologize, and fall silent. They also smiled more, a facial expression associated with subordinate status.

Much childhood play takes place in same-sex groups. It is an accepted part of boys' games that quarreling will occur. Boys frequently engage in fistfights and other scuffles to settle their disputes, then resume playing the game. Lasting hard feelings are rare. Later on, when they are lawyers or business executives, they will have no problem going for the jugular and then going for beers afterward (Heim, 1995). In contrast, when quarrels erupt during girls' games, play is most often terminated (Lever, 1976). But stopping the game without resolving the dispute may leave lingering resentments. These feelings may be expressed in a passive-aggressive way, such as two girls whispering together behind another girl's back, or several playmates deciding to shun one particular girl, the scapegoat of the conflict. There are hurt feelings about the ruptured relationships. I watched these dynamics in little girls' play closely when my daughter was younger. In the threesome of Shana, Vanessa, and Whitney, who went through preschool and the early grades together, Shana and Vanessa would gang up on Whitney, then Vanessa and Whitney would oust Shana, then Whitney and Shana would give the silent treatment to Vanessa, and so on, in ever-shifting triangles that conformed perfectly to Murray Bowen's theory. When it was my daughter Shana in tears over the latest tiff among the girls, I would encourage assertive, direct expression of her anger to her friends. But I was not successful in bringing about healthier resolution of conflict among the three over the long haul.

During adolescence, studies show that both the causes and the direction of anger expression are different for boys and girls. Adolescent females become angry because of interpersonal experiences and turn their anger inwardly, whereas males get angry in situations of performance evaluation and direct their anger outwardly (Stapley & Haviland, 1989). In a study of our own (Kollar, Groer, Thomas, & Cunningham, 1991), girls were especially anger-prone when someone tried to take advantage of their friendship. During adolescence the traditional sex-typed expectations of boys and girls become even more pronounced. Parents, teachers, and peers exert powerful pressures that are difficult to resist. Girls' anger expression is discouraged by a mechanism called invalidation (Crawford, Kippax, Onyx, Gault, & Benton, 1990). In other words, their anger is simply trivialized ("You're so cute when you're angry") or labeled as inappropriate ("What's wrong with you? Can't you be a good sport?"). As a result, a girl may question her own judgment of an incident or be ashamed of her outburst.

Brown and Gilligan (1992) conducted a 5-year study of the transition from girlhood to adolescence, documenting a kind of "psychological foot-binding" that took place over time. During the study, nearly 100 girls were interviewed yearly. At younger ages girls could speak about angry feelings. However, under enormous pressure to become "perfect girls" who were quiet, calm, and kind, the girls stopped expressing feelings such as anger by adolescence. They wanted to be popular and preserve relationships. Many of the girls seemed to be confused about whether anger really exists and whether they were really feeling angry. Adolescence was a time of repression of the self and the emotions, to avoid negative repercussions from other people.

What Brown and Gilligan described are the devastating effects of learning to be "feminine": of valuing others before oneself, responding to the opinions of others, fostering the well-being of others, and silencing one's own voice. Although there is a widespread myth that such self-sacrifice is an innate female virtue, it is clear that this is learned behavior. Learning to be "masculine" can be just as detrimental for subsequent emotional health. The aggressiveness that boys are encouraged to display does not serve them well as adults, when talking about feelings would be more appropriate than punching out walls or other people. Research on adults consistently shows that men are more likely to behave aggressively than women (Barefoot et al., 1991; Deffenbacher, 1994; Eagly & Steffen, 1986).

One authority who has studied aggression for 20 years (Campbell, 1993) contends that aggression feels good to men because it confers the reward of power and control over others. There is pride in a man's voice when he announces, "I told that SOB off" or "I punched him out." Loud cursing is the norm in many male-dominated workplaces, not only between peers but also directed at secretaries, receptionists, and messengers. For women, aggression does not feel good because it means failure of self-control—and guilt about the distress of the person who got the brunt of the attack. When women do become aggressive, their behavior isn't particularly effective in getting them what they want and need. For example, a woman who expresses anger to a spouse or lover may be told to calm down, take a tranquilizer, or get some therapy, continuing the invalidation she experienced in girlhood. She may retreat to more indirect methods of conveying her feelings, such as raising her eyebrows, sighing pointedly, or shaking her head, all of which are more common in women than in men (Deffenbacher, 1995a). Because aggression doesn't work effectively for them, most women just don't employ it very much. There is another reason why women are less aggressive: Such behavior may place them in danger. Retaliation in the form of sexual or physical assault is all too common.

Obviously, what we've covered so far is the effect of traditional gender role socialization. And it's quite clear that neither men's nor women's culturally assigned emotional behaviors serve them well. To what extent do most adults still conform to what they learned while growing up? Certainly, there can be "masculine" women and "feminine" men as well as androgynous individuals with some characteristics of both. What we've said about anger behavior applies to the extent that you behave in accordance with society's gender-specific rules. While adult men and women do not differ in the frequency of anger arousal (Averill, 1982), high scorers on masculine gender role identity express more anger and high scorers on femininity suppress more of it, regardless of actual biological sex (Kopper & Epperson, 1991).

As Averill (1982) argued persuasively, emotions are socially constituted syndromes that cannot be understood without consideration of the social context. Angry women threaten the status quo in a patriarchal society, so their anger is restricted in all societies where the military, industry, government, science community, and universities are in male hands. A 1993 United Nations Human Development Report found that there is still no country that treats its women as well as its men (cited in "The War Against Women," 1994). Where women still have lower status, power, and sense of self-worth than men, they must depend on men and others who are more powerful for approval. Consequently, they learn to be highly sensitive to nonverbal cues and hide their own emotional reactions to avoid antagonizing those in positions of dominance over them (Bernardez, 1987; Miller, 1983). In the words of Fiske (1993), "The powerless attend to the powerful who control their outcomes" (p. 621).

Women in our own study (Thomas et al., in press) had learned their early lessons well, as shown in these excerpts from the data:

> *If I got mad, I might say something off the wall that would hack everybody off and make a situation worse.*
> *It's better to go along with whatever's going on, if something's not immoral, than to push the issue.*
> *I try not to say things because I don't want things to escalate.*
> *I don't want to be known as a person who's hard to get along with, fussy and that kind of stuff.*

There is some evidence that younger women are more likely to express their anger forthrightly than midlife or older women, perhaps reflecting changes in societal norms (Thomas, 1997b). Today's 20-year-old woman watched television shows in the 1970s that featured aggressive heroines such as Wonder Woman and the Bionic Woman. One researcher (Huesmann, cited in Seppa, 1996) had assessed TV viewing habits of young girls between 1977 and 1979, and subsequently assessed their aggressive behavior as adults between 1992 and 1995, finding a significant correlation. Age differences in anger expression were found among 6 cohorts in the Women's Anger Study (Thomas, 1993b), with those 55 and older scoring highest on suppression of anger and the youngest cohort (age 34 or younger) scoring highest on anger frequency, angry thoughts, and anger vented outwardly. However, young women, like their older counterparts, remain hesitant to express their anger with lovers and spouses for fear of relationship loss (Asher & Hilton, 1996; Thomas, 1997b).

If you think that gendered rules for emotional expression have lessened sufficiently, think again. I would like to think so myself, but the longitudinal study by Brown and Gilligan (1992) of developing girls is not encouraging. One of our youngest Women's Anger Study participants, a 21-year-old, had this to say:

> *A lot of women my age are very very hesitant about . . . being angry, and even when we are angry . . . we want peace more than we want to actually express our anger and have somebody have to deal with it. Because then we have to deal with it too. It's a lot easier just to suppress it and not make anybody unhappy, and not have to deal with a confrontation, which bothers me. [This] makes me angry at myself.*

Boys are still being told that aggression is manly. While thumbing through *Time* magazine recently, I came across an essay that caught my attention. It was a father's advice to his son on the occasion of high school graduation. Its style was reminiscent of the best-selling *Life's Little Instruction Book.* (Brown, 1992). The son was being advised to vote, get a dog, do his own laundry, and so forth. But what struck me was the father's advice about fighting: *"If you find yourself in a fight"* (which I thought was a curious way to begin: how does a young man just *find* himself in a fight?) *"when you hit back, hit hard. Pick your time and place, and nuke 'em. Do not worry about making enemies. The right enemy will be a sign that you're growing up and that God loves you"* (Rosenblatt, 1997, p. 90). As long as fathers are telling their sons to "nuke 'em" and to consider accruing enemies as a badge of manly maturity, we are going to have a violent world.

What we learn while growing up, we carry into the workplace with us. Which brings us back to the world of nursing and the emotions flying about us as we do our jobs every day. Our phenomenological studies of anger in male and female nurses (Brooks et al., 1996; Smith et al., 1996) revealed commonalities as well as some interesting gender differences. Common to all narratives was the hostile work environment. Whether they were male or female, the nurses graphically described a virtual war zone in which they were frequently under assault by managers, peers, physicians, and patients. They spoke of anger as a weapon and a shield to defend against the assaults. A striking number of military metaphors ("on the firing line") and similes ("it's like an armed camp") appeared in the data:

> *I become very fatigued by having to do all these battles.*
> *I was getting flak.*

I went in with loaded guns.
You have to fight for what you get.
I was an easy target.
We feel sabotaged.
I see this real resistance and this real territorial stand.
We really don't know how to fight back.
There is character assassination.
You have to work close and not kill each other.
It's as though if you are the least bit quiet, gentle, or nonassertive, you're going to get your head knocked off.

MALE NURSES AND ANGER

In response to the hostile work environment, both male and female nurses often felt powerless. Their environment caused them to be on the defensive. But the anger of the men was much more intense and included elements of aggression. They used words such as *rage* and *red fury* that were never used by the women. One man said, "You get so angry, your face turns red, almost as if you are blowing fire out of your nose." Male nurses acknowledged violent impulses—"What I would really like to do is slap somebody, just reach up and slap them real good;" "You just want to hit or shake someone;" "I wanted to kill her"—although they did not act on these impulses. The men thought of violent actions most often when they were being attacked by a physician or supervisor in the presence of other people.

What do male nurses do with their virulent anger? Based on our interview data (Brooks et al., 1996), isolation was the men's most common response to workplace anger. In the words of Mike Evans, "My way of handling it is to distance myself." Greg James stated, "I shut off everything around me. I turn it inward. I have a sense of being completely alone." Male nurses isolated themselves not only to avoid an episode of uncontrolled anger, but also after expressing their anger or receiving angry attacks from others. Crying was viewed as a loss of control, and when a loss of control seemed imminent, the men chose to remove themselves from the situation. For example, Ron said, "I had to leave after that. I just had to leave."

I find it very understandable that men in nursing would choose to distance themselves after experiencing anger. Generally speaking, men in our society are more likely to internalize their emotional distress, whereas women often seek solace and support from others when they are upset. Men in nursing may be doubly reluctant to reveal emotional distress to their female coworkers because of past experiences of gender discrimination. However, by isolating themselves, men remove any possibility of receiving empathy, support, or affirmation from female peers or supervisors. Sadly, the men in our study often told of relationships with colleagues that were completely severed because anger was not worked through. For example, Bob Hayes purposely chose to work a different shift after an angry experience with a female nurse. Before the anger incident, the two had been good friends and had always taken their lunch or break together. By changing shifts, he succeeded in avoiding her, but he described his shifts as "long and lonely."

Some male nurses described a deliberate controlled form of anger that was not often evident in our data from female nurses. This form of anger was called "corrective" or "appropriate" and was used to gain attention or to be heard. In the words of Tom Parker, "Anger can be a driving force to open up a problem." He went on to explain: "I learned to use anger in a very controlled sense . . . in a way that would make a point . . . drive my point home." This use of anger as a tool is healthy. Women in nursing should marshal it for their use as well.

FEMALE NURSES AND ANGER

When I, along with my research team, first grappled with the data from female nurses, I was inclined to agree with Germaine Greer (1991), who contended that "despite the best efforts of feminists to awaken women's anger and to turn their hostility outward so that it becomes a force for social change rather than the procreator of symptoms, we have failed (p. 120)." Although female nurses had no hesitation in pouring out their pent-up feelings to our research team, they had not expressed their ire directly to the people who provoked them. They were waiting for others to rescue them, to take care of them, and to make things right. Although overt anger erupted in some situations, more often women's anger was expressed indirectly in passive-aggressive fashion or turned inward on the self. When anger exploded in screaming, the female nurses sought to disown their emotion. This account of an anger incident sounded much like a dissociative episode:

My mind's racing. I'm just coming out of myself, and when I come back I just sometimes look and I can't believe I've done that, like that's really not me. I let somebody else provoke me into behaving in a way that I wouldn't normally act, that's not really acceptable.

Nurses' reactions to overt anger expression are consistent with the rules of feminine behavior. When Fran blows up, she feels ineffective, experiences guilt, and views herself as less than professional. Ann refers to herself as a "bitch" when she expresses her anger. Sally says she feels embarrassed. Even the reviewers of our manuscript about female nurses' anger recoiled in dismay at its "ugliness." One of the reviewers admitted that she "cringed" at the words used by our study participants and found them "unbecoming for professionals." This reviewer wanted the data sanitized, removing all profanity. I am grateful that the editor did not ask us to do this, because it would not have been ethical to alter the research data.

The data indicate that female nurses are inhibited in effective use of anger by their gender role socialization. Maybe it's time for a "killing." Author Virginia Woolf found it necessary to "kill off" the nagging internal voice of the ideal feminine homemaker so that she could go beyond that role and become a writer. As Woolf sat at her table to compose a literary critique, she could hear "the Angel in the House" admonishing her that she should flatter the author and never let anyone know that she had a sharp mind of her own. The "Angel" wanted her to be ever-charming, sympathetic, and tender, as she had been socialized in Victorian England to be. But Woolf could not write literary criticism within these rigid confines of gender, and so she killed the "Angel," for "had I not killed her she would have killed me" (Woolf, cited in Levinson, 1996, p. 50).

Female nurses were more likely to verbalize anger to advocate for their patients than to fight for their own rights. Likewise, in the Women's Anger Study we found that women could assert themselves on behalf of their children, but not achieve relationship reciprocity with their spouses. Women generally do not have a sense that their anger can be used to good effect in their relationships. Whether they hold anger in or vent it outwardly, they still do not get the desired result and end up feeling that the attempt was futile. They feel powerless to get others to change their behavior. They wonder why their anger is not efficacious. A participant in the Women's Anger Study said that her attempts to get members of her family to pick up their strewn belongings were "fruitless. . . . I'll say it and it's just like it goes in one ear and out the other. I'm not stating it right or something. It doesn't work" (Thomas et al., in press). Here is an example of the same bewilderment and futility from a nurse in my anger workshop:

I work nights. One of the RNs on days is always late. She is a great person. We both graduated from nursing school together many years ago. She is slightly crippled and uses this to get away with always being late. After a 12-hour shift my crew and I are quite eager to get home. We have teased her, begged her, threatened her, reported her, but nothing has worked. I was angry, I am angry, but it appears that nothing can be done.

These women have not yet learned that when the transgressor does not and will not change, what they need to do is affirm their anger as justified but move on to problem-solving. An asset for women is their willingness to confide in a friend or relative when they are upset. Unlike the male nurses who isolate themselves, females do seek a listening ear. As we discussed in Chapter 4, talking out a problem elicits empathy and feedback. Furthermore, as you review the anger incident, you may develop insight into the dynamics of the interaction. Ideas to solve the problem are often generated as well. It's the same principle by which psychotherapy works. Our male colleagues in nursing could benefit from allowing themselves to reveal their pain and vulnerability to another nurse, just as females could benefit from learning to use anger as a driving force to open up a problem.

TOWARD TRANSCENDING GENDER ROLE SOCIALIZATION

It's clear that both female and male nurses have a bit of work to do. To be an emotionally healthy adult requires transcending the restrictions of masculine and feminine gender roles and developing a diverse repertoire of emotion behaviors. We have all been constrained by what we learned while growing up, but it's not too late to chuck the rules. Individuals who develop a style that includes behaviors not usually associated with their gender socialization are more creative, flexible, integrative, and spontaneous (Cummings, 1995). Throughout this book, we present new approaches that you can try. However, once you have moved beyond rigid conformity to gender rules, other obstacles to healing and wholeness remain. One such obstacle, and a very significant one, is painful trauma in your past, which is the topic of our next chapter.

8

Overcoming the Legacy of a Painful or Abusive Past

> Anger is healthy, while resentment and hate are
> detrimental. . . . Anger is fresh, expansive, active,
> constructive, and varies with changes in the situation.
> Resentment and hate are past-oriented. . . . They remain
> and remain, working chiefly on and against oneself.
>
> Eugene Gendlin

Many nurses are mired in resentment about the past: pain inflicted by a mother who was critical, a father who was never around, a brother or sister who was the favorite and got more "goodies," a lover who dumped them for someone else, a friend who turned out to be a traitor, a lost educational or work opportunity. While their anger may be entirely justifiable—at least, initially—it begins to affect their mental health when it's chronic and corrosive. Old angers often mingle with new ones in a multilayered amalgam, hurtful incident piled upon other hurtful incidents, until there is so much bad feeling that there's hardly any room for joy. Remember the woman who talked about her unexpressed anger that "rolled up into a big ball"? To refresh your memory, here's what she said:

> *It's like you build up so much anger inside or resentment towards somebody without really sitting down and talking about the problem that it just rolls up into a big ball and you're not even sure what it's really about. And then you have to take that ball apart again in little sections and you've got to ask questions and poke places that are really deep and hurt you sometimes.*

This chapter is about unraveling your ball of anger and taking it apart, bit by bit, so that you can overcome the legacy of a painful or abusive past. Yes, when you poke tender places, there will still be some twinges of pain. If you have experienced severe trauma, you may need to work with a therapist while you unravel your ball of anger. Because your greatest pain has been inflicted in relationships, healing must also take place in a relationship. Throughout life, we work through unfinished business from old relationships in new ones. Not only therapists but also lovers, spouses, friends, and teachers help us to heal. With or without a therapist, letting go of angry feelings may seem to be a formidable undertaking. One of our study participants who admitted having a lot of stored anger asked:

How do you get back to point A from point D? Because I've passed B and C, you know. It's like I'm way out here, how do I get myself back over there? When you've got so much anger built up, how do you get back? How do you get rid of 20 years of your father and your husband and your mother and relationships that you probably shouldn't even care about? How do I get rid of all this? I don't know.

The word *heal* is defined in the dictionary as "to become well or whole again, to restore . . . to health . . . to cause painful emotions to be no longer grievous." How can we reach a place of peace where painful emotions are no longer "grievous"? There are many paths to emotional healing. Bringing long-buried material to consciousness, developing insight into painful events, talking with someone who cares are just a few of the ways that have proved to be helpful. Other avenues to healing will be explored throughout this chapter.

Carl Jung gave the world an enormously helpful, optimistic psychology that emphasized the self-healing psyche: We must look within to discover its wisdom. Many Jungian analysts believe that the healing process can be facilitated by keeping a journal. There are many ways to do this, from the complex method recommended by therapist Ira Progoff (1975) to simple stream-of-consciousness musings jotted down in a notepad. I have kept a journal all my life and find this activity invaluable in processing events and gaining self-knowledge. It is especially useful every 5 years or so to pull out some old volumes (my books are all sizes and colors, heaped in a big box in the closet) to see what I was dealing with, and how I understood it, at various times. Working through pain is a lifelong process. My personal growth has been like a spiral, sometimes looping back, then going forward a bit, rather than a linear trajectory.

Throughout my life I have spiraled back to revisit some of the same painful events, such as the death of my parents when I was very young. But as I review the journals, I find evidence of progress in my perspective on the events. Each time I let go of a little more resentment, and in so doing, open myself to greater joy. The cruel reality of the events never changes, but my view of them does.

If you would like to start keeping a journal, I have only one recommendation: Write in it regularly. Some authorities specify a certain number of pages each day, but I am not so rigidly prescriptive. I do not even insist that you write a journal entry every day. But there must be a rhythm of some kind, a process so routinized that thoughts and feelings flow quickly onto the page before they can be censored and "cleaned up" to look respectable. Your journal is for no eyes but yours, so do not sanitize its contents. You can record dreams in your journal too, if you like. Dreams are messages from yourself to yourself, delivered when you are psychologically ready to receive and integrate them. When regularly recorded, reflected on, and understood, dreams transmit wisdom from deep in the psyche to your conscious mind.

Marion Woodman, a Jungian analyst, has recommended keeping a journal as a way of facing your "swamp of anguish and aggression":

> *The daily journal is like a mirror. When we first look into it, the blank pages stare back with ominous emptiness. But if we keep looking and trusting in what [Rainer Maria] Rilke calls "the possibility of being," gradually we begin to see the face that is looking back at us. If we stand naked, the mirror reflects things as they are. There is more to the mirror than reflection. The long hours of sitting alone stripping off the self-deceptions, the artificial self-pity, the self-inflicted maiming, build the . . . connection between the conscious and unconscious worlds in a way that connects both. With the mirror, we go through, we take our reality into another world, the world of the unconscious, and find a relationship to our own soul. Journal writing is a way of taking responsibility for finding out who I AM. Facing our dark sides is painful. It is easier to turn away from our own swamp of anguish and aggression and say "It doesn't matter. I've got friends. I'm well adjusted to my job. Everyone likes me." The mirror will not let us off the hook. It says "It does matter. If you're not experiencing life it does matter. Where was your own laughter today? Where are your tears?" (Woodman, 1982, pp. 99, 101)*

The answer to Woodman's questions about your absent laughter and tears may lie in traumatic events that caused you to shut down your emotions. For some of you, the event may be the loss of a loved one, and you are still numb because of grief. Perhaps you have lost a parent, a spouse, a child. The word *bereavement* comes from the Old English *beroafian*, which means "to rob, to plunder, or to dispose." Death robs us of a loved one, often precipitously. Snatched away is a person who made you feel special, who cared about what you were doing, who cheered you on to do great things. I first learned what this searing pain is like when my father left for the office one day and never came home again. Perhaps you learned when you lost a child, and had to bury all the shining dreams you once had for him. For a few weeks after a death, there are calls and cards, and hastily proffered pies and tuna casseroles from people who won't come inside ("Gotta run; call me if you need anything"), and then the house is quiet. Very quiet. You are bereft. Healing during bereavement is a long-term process. The anguish seems interminable. In our world of instant coffee, instant communication, and instant relief of discomfort, no one has patience with long-term processes like mourning. So you go back to work and try to act "normal" even though you feel hollow inside. After awhile, no one mentions your loss anymore. After all, you should be "all better" by now. It's been 2 years, hasn't it?

Or perhaps your hurt and anger are encapsulated, smouldering inside you because of the horror of physical or sexual abuse. Perhaps you were abusively disciplined "for your own good." Perhaps your daddy came into your room at night and did things that you didn't understand. If these things happened to you, you are not alone. The statistics are staggering. According to Holz (1994), 45% of health care providers were victims of abuse during childhood. One in 4 girls and 1 in 7 boys are sexually abused in some way before their 18th birthday (Browne & Finkelhor, 1986). One study of undergraduate nursing students at a major university found that 47% of the females and 38% of the males had had one or more unwanted sexual experiences in childhood (Rew & Christian, 1993). Nurses who had experienced childhood sexual abuse revealed its effects on their personal and professional lives in interviews conducted by a Toronto research team (Gallop, McKeever, Toner, Lancee, & Lueck, 1995):

I think it definitely has affected . . . the way I act sexually. . . . I'm very skeptical that there are really good loving relationships.
[I have] difficulty trusting [a] male staff physician and one or two coworkers. . . .
[I spent] many years as a timid, unsure, nonassertive doormat, afraid of ridicule or being ignored. [I] don't want to be noticed.

*I'm a total wimp. . . . I can allow myself to be manipulated. I can allow
myself to have other people do the choosing and stuff like that.
I think the abuse contributed to my feeling, kind of . . . less than worthy.*

The nursing profession includes not only survivors of childhood
abuse but also many women who have experienced partner abuse as
adults. One in every 3 women in the United States experiences abuse
from a male partner at least once during her lifetime (Straus & Gelles,
1987). In a recent survey of obstetrical nurses working in hospitals, private offices, and community health, 31% reported abuse of either self
or a close family member (Moore, Parsons, & Zaccaro, 1997). Tragi-
cally, some nurses have experienced abuse as both children and adults.

Although there is not much in the literature about it, nurses also receive abuse from patients. The assault rate in health care facilities is increasing (Lanza et al., 1996), but nurses underreport patient assaults
and receive little support from their colleagues and management
(Lanza, 1983). Roberts (1991) contended that assault against nurses in
the workplace is silenced, just as assault within families is. To shed some
light on the experience of abused nurses, Roberts conducted a qualitative study of 12 female nurses who had been assaulted by patients. All of
the nurses reported strong emotional responses to the assault (anger
being the most common) and long-term consequences for their job
performance. They believed that management blamed them for the assault, either explicitly or implicitly. They found themselves labeled as
"the nurse who got hit." Their institutions seemed to view violence
against staff as part of the job. Lack of support by the institutions and
the police outraged the women. Management seldom supported prose-
cution of the attacker, and the nurses were reluctant to proceed with
legal action on their own. Coping strategies of the nurses were mainly
avoidant: minimizing, denying, and forgetting about the assault. One
nurse intensified her efforts to look like a good, unblemished and virtuous nurse. She said that in the months following the attack, she
bought "the whitest pair of stockings and the whitest pair of shoes" so
that she would look like the "quintessential nurse." The traumatic experience of these nurses indicates that much needs to be done to reduce not only the violence itself but also its damaging sequelae.

There is another kind of abuse, a kind that leaves no visible black
eyes or bruises but deeply scars a person's soul. Verbal abuse can take
many forms: ridicule, disparagement, criticism, accusations, threats,
name-calling, sarcastic "humor" that isn't funny, and the cold silence
that conveys rejection. Many nurses have experienced this kind of
abuse from a parent or lover. It can take place at the job site too, as

shown in our research data (see Chapter 5 regarding verbal abuse by physicians). One of the devastating effects of the abuse is an insidious change in the victim's self-concept. She (or he) begins to internalize the criticism and accept its validity: "After all, he knows me better than anyone, and if he thinks I am (unlovable, dumb, unattractive, clumsy, incompetent, etc.), then it must be true." The abuse is usually kept from friends and relatives because the victim is ashamed, so there is no one to provide a reality check and corrective feedback. To complicate matters further, many abusers are socially charming and display their meanness only in private. Thus, there are no witnesses.

The consequences of abuse resemble the posttraumatic stress syndrome (PTSD) common to survivors of disasters and combat: denial, confusion, fear, nightmares, flashbacks, and psychological numbing. But there are some important distinctions: Neither disaster victims nor soldiers were harmed by individuals they loved and trusted. Furthermore, survivors of disasters and wars do not blame themselves for what happened, as abuse victims tend to do. Finally, survivors of disasters and wars can usually talk about their traumatic experiences without shame. In contrast, experiences of abuse are often kept secret: I have worked with and taught many victims of abuse who had never told anyone before.

The literature tends to emphasize the devastating sequelae of abuse rather than the potential for healing. Persons who have been abused tend to distrust others, fear those with greater power, and have lower self-esteem. They are at high risk for depression, substance abuse, and other crippling aftereffects. They may commit or attempt to commit suicide. But we also know that countless victims of abuse go on to lead satisfying and productive lives. The scars from abuse can, and do, heal. If you have been abused and are still suffering some of the sequelae, please get into therapy now. Know that the violence, whether physical, sexual, or verbal, was not your fault. Start on the healing path.

Therapist Carl Rogers used to tell a story about the potatoes stored during the winter in the cellar of his home. Toward the one tiny window in the cellar, long spindly sprouts of the potatoes would strain to reach light. Rogers saw many of his patients in this way: in a dark cellar of fear, sadness, or self-loathing, yet nevertheless still seeking the light and growing in the process of doing so. I think that all of us are a bit like Carl Rogers's potatoes. Getting to the light—being enlightened, fully aware—takes time. Lillian Hellman explained the process:

Old paint on canvas, as it ages, sometimes becomes transparent. When that happens it is possible, in some pictures, to see the original lines: a tree will show through a woman's dress, a child makes way for a dog, a large boat is no longer on an open sea. That is called pentimento because the painter "repented," changed his mind. Perhaps it would be as well to say that the old conception, replaced by a later choice, is a way of seeing and then seeing again. (Hellman, 1973, p. 3)

STRENGTHENING PERSONAL BOUNDARIES

Strengthening personal boundaries is a necessary step for many nurses who are trying to overcome the legacy of a painful or abusive past. Boundaries are the demarcation lines that separate me from you. They refer to your physical body and personal space as well as to your psyche and emotions. If you are overly compliant with others' opinions, fear disagreement, and lack the ability to say what you really feel—even when treated badly—you have some boundary problems. Difficulties with boundaries are common in individuals who grew up in families where

- parents discounted a child's feelings and needs
- independence was thwarted, while dependence or clinging behavior was rewarded
- boundaries of the family members were blurred, distorted, nonexistent, or fragmented (e.g., in an alcoholic family)
- boundaries were disrespected or invaded for the sexual gratification of adults

You will need to work on development of a sense of yourself as strong and separate from others. Boundaries are vitally important to protect yourself from the emotions of others and to set limits on others who are mistreating you. Anger, when channeled into clear verbal messages, can be an excellent mechanism for protecting your boundaries. If you have started working with a therapist, he or she will help you strengthen your boundaries.

STRENGTHENING SELF-ESTEEM

In addition to strengthening your boundaries, it's time to work on strengthening your self-esteem. While the next few paragraphs may be useful to some male nurses reading this book, I must speak specifically to females for a bit. There's a good reason for doing so: The research consistently shows that the self-esteem of females is lower than that of males. This should not be surprising, given the pervasive devaluing of women in our society. Self-esteem is partly a function of the social relations and processes in which individuals are embedded. Women do not have as many sources of external validation as men do. The nurturing work they do—nursing, teaching, child care—is undervalued by society. Mary Catherine Bateson (1990) speaks of the "ingrained and disabling sense of inferiority" (p. 38) characteristic of American women. Although she is an accomplished professional woman, she confesses, "I have slighted my own value so often that it is hard to learn to take it seriously." (p. 40) Even the potent external validation of achieving great fame and influence does not always penetrate a woman's self-perception of her worth. Witness the shocking disclosure of influential feminist activist and writer Gloria Steinem regarding her own low self-esteem in her book *Revolution From Within: A Book of Self-Esteem* (1991). It goes to show that neither brilliance nor glamour nor renown guarantees a solid sense of personal worth.

Despite the advances over the past few decades as a result of the women's movement, in which Steinem played such a leading role, today's high school girls still a poorer self-image than their male counterparts. A recent survey sponsored by the American Association of University Women (Freiberg, 1991) showed that self-esteem of girls drops as they mature. Although about 60% of girls were confident in elementary school, by high school the percentage had declined to 29%. It's not a coincidence that the decrease in self-esteem occurs during those years that girls are under enormous pressure to be "perfect girls" and hide their true emotions so that they will be "popular," as documented in the longitudinal study conducted by Brown and Gilligan (1992). The "perfect girls" move into adulthood determined to be perfect wives and mothers, perfect professionals. Because perfection is an impossible goal, they are setting themselves up for failure and self-recrimination.

What is self-esteem? It's the degree to which we value ourselves, a judgment made largely on the basis of others' appraisals (especially those in our circle of intimates) and to a lesser extent on self-evaluation of our accomplishments. It's a view based in part on the way our parents treated us but modified by later life experiences. Those with lower self-esteem have often been the victims of physical or verbal abuse. Because they do not have a positive view of themselves, they are at the mercy of others' evaluation, increasing their risk of being taken advantage of in work situations (Gallop et al., 1995).

In the Women's Anger Study, our research team found that the lower the self-esteem, the higher a woman's tendency to anger easily (Saylor & Denham, 1993). Women with low self-esteem manage that anger more inappropriately too, stuffing it or lashing out at others. As we have seen in earlier chapters, these ways of managing anger further reinforce low self-esteem, perpetuating the cycle. When a woman stuffs her anger instead of telling others her honest feelings, she gets mad at herself for remaining silent. And when she lashes out, there's fallout in terms of damaged relationships, remorse, and guilt about the outburst. The woman feels isolated, inadequate, and misunderstood. Obviously, this cycle should be broken, but how?

The good news is that self-esteem is modifiable (Crouch & Straub, 1983). But to work on our self-esteem, we first have to develop a different mindset. Many of us think that displaying healthy self-esteem (looking and acting confident, being sure of ourselves, and remaining unapologetic about making reasonable requests or stating opinions) is unfeminine. We wouldn't want to be viewed as too forward, pushy, mannish, or lacking in proper humility. Sometimes when we tried to point out our accomplishment we received negative feedback from our peers or from persons in positions of dominance who preferred a more obsequious employee or lover. As part of our gender role socialization, we were taught to say instead, "Oh, it was really nothing," about our successes.

How can self-esteem be modified? First, engage in some reflection about the way you developed your view of yourself during childhood. Think back to childhood nicknames, interactions with parents, siblings, and playmates, times of performance evaluation such as bringing home your report card. What tapes are still playing over and over in your mind? Look at photo albums; talk to family members. In every family, someone is labeled the "ugly duckling" or the "black sheep." Was that you? If so, what were some of the smart and brave things that you did to make it through a childhood that was lonely or traumatic? Here are smart and brave things that you can do now.

Steps Toward Healing

1. Enlarge your sources of self-esteem. Some women limit the sources from which they seek validation to just one or two other people—perhaps just their husband or lover—so that the criticisms of these people are inordinately powerful. Find times to be with friends who enjoy your company, appreciate you, and verbally affirm your strengths. Consider a support group in which

members validate each other (as we talked about in an earlier chapter).

2. Validate yourself with positive self-talk. You already know how to give others praise and encouragement. Do the same for yourself. Focus on your strengths instead of your weaknesses. Affirm yourself for trying, making progress, taking risks to do things you never thought you could do. Congratulate yourself for being a member of a noble profession that provides an indispensable service to society. When you succeed at something, give yourself proper credit. Researchers have found that when women succeed, they call it luck; when women fail, they consider themselves stupid. In contrast, when men succeed, they give themselves credit; when they fail, they blame an outside source (Sanford & Donovan, 1985).

3. Consult the "wise woman" within. This is an imagery exercise that I have found very helpful when I work with women. To do the exercise, first become deeply relaxed. Unplug the phone, dim the lights, and seat yourself in a comfortable position. Close your eyes. Pay attention to your breathing for a few minutes. Imagine your body as hollow and allow each breath to fill your hollow body. When you are ready, let yourself become aware that you are not alone. With you is a wise woman who is concerned with your well-being. You can trust her. Make contact with this woman. Notice the love and wisdom with which you are surrounded. Tell your wise guide anything you wish. Ask her, "What do I need to do to feel better about myself?" Listen to the answers that emerge. Maintain an attitude of openness to her advice. After your imagery is finished, reflect quietly. What did she recommend?

Are you aware that the wise woman is really a part of yourself? Every one of us has something deep inside that knows our true nature and purpose in life. It has been called the Center. Carl Jung called it the greater Self. Here we depicted it as the archetypal figure of the wise woman. You may wish to conceptualize it in congruence with a particular religious orientation. The important thing is to gain access to your own inner wisdom and benefit from its guidance.

FORGIVING AND MOVING ON

But maybe, just maybe, forgiveness exists not to excuse the sinner but to heal those who suffered. This idea seems true and honest to me for this reason: As

Mama became less able to forgive my daddy, her anger grew like wildfire and began to burn us all. (Fowler, 1996, p. 105)

These words are taken from *Before Women Had Wings,* Connie May Fowler's story of her abusive and impoverished childhood. Her understanding of forgiveness is remarkable, given what she endured: the suicide of her father, the dreadful beatings from her alcoholic mother, and even being "jilted by Jesus." That she survived it all, and shares what she learned about forgiveness through her writing, is impressive evidence of human resilience. There is a wealth of wisdom about suffering, and transcending it, in literature, drama, and film. I have found exemplars such as Fowler's tremendously helpful in my own journey to healing.

I know firsthand that being able to forgive is an essential step in emotional healing. It accomplishes nothing to leave old wounds open so that new salt can inflame them from time to time. What does it mean to forgive? It does not mean condoning the hurtful actions of those who abandoned you or treated you badly. In fact, it is an important step to acknowledge that you deserved better treatment than you got. The next step is a conscious decision to relinquish the role of wronged victim. One lesson that I have learned through my clinical work and research is that the role of wronged victim serves no one well. As long as you define yourself as a victim, you are not free. Forgiveness is a way of freeing yourself so that the person who wronged you no longer has the power to define you. It is a way of releasing yourself from the anguish of your past life and moving on.

I spent my adolescent years bitter and alienated, acting out and being envious of others who had loving families and support. I could not imagine why I had ever been born. I was angry at life, angry at the world, and angry at God—if there was a God. In my distorted view, my misery was unique. What a life-changing event it was when I went to work at a hospital at the age of 15. My friend Judy, who wanted to be a nurse, had talked me into applying for a job with her at St. Joseph's Hospital. The hospital hired the two of us as nurses' aides on the 3-to-11 shift; we went to high school from 8 a.m. to 2 p.m., and then to the hospital to work. On our floor were young mothers dying of cancer, diabetics losing their legs—the gamut of gripping tragedy and human suffering. I had never thought about being a nurse, but working with these patients produced a dramatic change in my perspective and helped me to begin healing. Even as a nurses' aide with no training, I was able to provide comfort to people who hurt. It was deeply satisfying when I gave a patient a backrub and properly plumped each pillow, then tiptoed out as he quietly went to sleep.

Later on, when I became a psychiatric nurse, I moved a bit farther on the healing path as I listened to my patients describe every kind of abuse and atrocity imaginable. So many of them had endured far more pain and trauma in their early years than I. How could I hold on to my old resentment? When you peer into the hearts and minds of others, you learn that every family is somewhat dysfunctional, and every person is a bit neurotic. Nobody has it easy. Loneliness, failure, shame, loss, betrayal, confusion—they're all there, in each and every human psyche.

The world breaks everyone, and afterward many are strong at the broken places. (Hemingway, cited in Viorst, 1986, p. 260)

Life will send us, not what we want, but what we need in order to grow. (Sanford, 1977, p. 20)

Although it is standard advice in many nursing texts to tell people to "find meaning" in their adversity, I believe that some of the blows from life are never fully comprehensible. We often brood in anger over unfairness: Why me? Why now? What did I do to deserve this? Answers are slow in coming, and we may never find a satisfactory answer. Kierkegaard pointed out that "life can only be understood backwards; but it must be lived forwards." I don't expect to ever understand everything. Perhaps mental peace is ultimately a matter of becoming reconciled to mystery. I strongly believe that for mental peace and healing we must forgive those who played a part in the pain of the past. I like these two quotes from Colgrove et al. (1991):

To forgive does not just mean to pardon, it means to let go. (p. 148)

If you are tied to a rock that is pulling you down in the water, all you have to do is forgive it . . . and swim toward the light. (p. 148)

Old anger, bitterness, and sadness can indeed be heavy rocks pulling you down. Why not let go and forgive? How liberating it is to unpack some of the heavy emotional baggage and forgive the parents who neglected you, the friends who let you down, the lovers who fell out of love with you. Forgiving can be done verbally, either with the person who wronged you or with a counselor, symbolically through a healing ritual, or in writing—a letter, a poem, perhaps a journal entry. Novelist Connie May Fowler views her writing as the vehicle for forgiving her deceased parents. Jack Kornfield recommends a formal forgiveness meditation, using these words: "There are many ways I have been wounded and hurt, abused and abandoned, by others in thought, word, or deed, knowingly or unknowingly. . . . To the extent that I am ready, I offer them forgiveness. I have carried this pain in my heart too long. For this reason, to those who have caused me harm, I offer you my forgiveness. I forgive you" (Kornfield, 1993, p. 286). The meditation is repeated until you can feel a release in your heart. Reciting the psalms is another way for you to give up anger and move toward healing (Saussy, 1995). When those who wronged you are deceased or far away, you can still forgive them, because forgiveness is something that happens within you.

Many people benefit from healing rituals. For example, you might burn, cut up, or throw away pictures or other items that evoke painful memories. Or you could make something new: a piece of pottery, a painting of your family. There is a painting by Joan Snyder in the National Museum of Women in the Arts entitled "Can We Turn Our Rage to Poetry?" The title makes me think of wonderful poets who have done so: Marge Piercy, Robert Bly, to name only two. While not all of us are blessed with the talents of a painter or a poet, there are a number of ways to creatively release anger and pain. You can even bring a bit of humor to your healing ritual. An acquaintance of mine who was newly divorced threw an "Un-Wedding Party." She served her guests 7-Up (then being touted in ads as the "un-cola"), threw rice at them, and gave them "gifts" of marriage-related memorabilia she no longer wanted in her house. The piece de résistance was a glorious lopsided un-wedding cake of many layers, with globs of cherries cascading down its sides. By announcing her new single status with humor and style, this woman put the heartbreak of a failed marriage behind her. We cheered her ability to forgive her ex-husband and move on with her life.

Taking actions to help others in pain also promotes healing (Montgomery, 1991). When Rubin (1996) studied individuals who had transcended a difficult past, she found a strong sense of mission in their stories, a commitment to something beyond their personal interests. They were determined to use their painful experiences of the past to change the present for others. Some people who have been abused choose an occupation like nursing or social work or volunteer their time to work in shelters for the abused: *"I now work in community mental health, do counseling and am very active in the women's movement fighting sexual, physical, and emotional abuse. I have done workshops on violence against women and supervise counselors who do this work"* (nurse interviewed by Gallop et al., 1995, p. 142).

This nurse is what Carl Jung called a "wounded healer." In mythology, the wounded healer is represented in Chiron, the centaur-teacher of Asclepius. But we need not dust off our knowledge of Greek mythology because examples are all around us in health care settings: recovering alcoholics who counsel other alcoholics, cancer survivors who visit patients facing surgery, pediatricians who had been sickly children themselves and now give compassionate care to children. How does working with other wounded individuals assist in healing our own wounds? First, it alters our perspective on our own suffering, redeeming the pain of the past because we can see that healing gifts have resulted from that pain. Second, when we minister to others in a loving way, we are loving ourselves as well—binding our wounds, so to speak. If you have been denying your woundedness, I encourage you to claim it, for you will be a better healer.

RESILIENCE, COHERENCE, AND THE RIVER

Thankfully, there is a new emphasis in the psychiatric/mental health literature on the human capacity for resilience and victory over "handicapping" traumas and tragedies (O'Leary & Ickovics, 1994; Rubin, 1996). A large study of adults, ages 23 to 87, showed that most people who endure divorce, the death of a loved one, or other major misfortunes emerge stronger and better able to cope with subsequent events in their lives (Aldwin, Sutton, & Lachman, 1996). There have been other important studies on resilience that debunk the old notions of inevitable emotional scarring or psychopathology from losses, broken homes, poverty, and the like. We can take heart from the following:

- *Seventy-five percent of the children of alcoholics do not become alcoholics (Wolin, cited in Secunda, 1994)*
- *Women who had childhood stresses, such as divorce or remarriage of their parents or death of a loved one, are less likely to become depressed when they face distress-provoking situations in adulthood (Forest, 1991).*
- *In a study of over 400 famous men and women of the 20th century, researchers found that 75% of them had been highly stressed in childhood by physical handicaps or defects, broken homes, or economic deprivation (Goertzel & Goertzel, 1962).*
- *Twenty-nine percent of Israeli women who survived the horror of World War II concentration camps, years as displaced persons, and three wars in Israel were found to be emotionally healthy in midlife (Antonovsky, 1987).*

The last-cited study of Israeli women proved to be a dramatic turning point in researcher Aaron Antonovsky's work as a medical sociologist.

Even though the percentage of concentration camp survivors in good mental health was not large, Antonovsky was impressed by the resilience and strength they had demonstrated. He wanted to know what distinguished those survivors from others who were overwhelmed by stress and negative emotions, so he embarked on further studies of men and women to find out. What Antonovsky found is something that he calls the "sense of coherence," which is a feeling of confidence that one can manage and find meaning, even in chaos. People who had a strong sense of coherence responded: *"You have to take life as it comes"; "When something terrible happens, people look for someone to blame. But I don't; absolutely not"; "I never felt that I was getting a raw deal"; "I decided you just have to overcome; I won't let myself be broken."*

In contrast, people with a weak sense of coherence said: *"All of life is a constant battle"; "All of life is full of problems; only in dying [are] there no problems"; "Everyone screwed me"; "They ruined my whole life"; "Things are rough; I don't have any faith left in anyone"; "It's all because my father died when I was a kid and I kept wandering around"* (Antonovsky, 1987, pp. 69–74).

The difference in the two mental attitudes is striking, isn't it? The people who had a strong "sense of coherence" have gotten beyond anger and blame. They were able to persist during periods of suffering and darkness in their lives. They are healed. You too can be healed. Wash away your wounds and bear no scars, as depicted in the river metaphor from David Reynolds's book *Water Bears No Scars* (1987):

> *A rushing stream of water flows around the obstacles that stand in its way. It doesn't stop to dwell on the injuries sustained by a projecting rock or a submerged log. It keeps moving toward its goal, encountering each difficulty as it appears, responding actively, then moving along downstream. It washes away its own wounds in its present purposefulness. The water bears no scars.*

9

Caring for the Self

Let me put you on hold—there's an urgent e-mail
coming in, and, uh-oh, just a second, somebody's at
my office door. No, I haven't graded your paper yet.
I thought that I might get to finish it and read my mail
while I ate my lunch. But it's almost 2:00 and I haven't
had time for lunch yet, and I've got a meeting at
2:30. Why didn't I think to buy a cup of yogurt this
morning? Guess I'll have to get something out of the
snack machine. I've got a few minutes between my
meeting and my night class, so I promise I'll finish your
paper and put it in your mailbox before I leave.

Vignette from a typical day at the university for me

The American Holistic Nurses Association says that practicing nursing requires nurses to integrate self-care in their own lives. While I heartily agree, I know how difficult it is to take care of our own needs in our hectic work environments, whether they are health departments, clinics, hospitals, or nursing schools. How many times do you skip lunch or postpone taking a break?

The majority of nurses in a large national study perceived their work environments as "constraining," in that they could not properly meet their physical needs for breaks and meals or their professional needs for autonomy (Carlson-Catalano, 1990). The problem, of course, is not just the demands of the work environment. It's the tendency of nurses to allow themselves to be engulfed in the needs of others, consequently neglecting their own.

Nurse historians have provided interesting glimpses of the phenomenon in the early days of the profession. For example, consider the

California debate in the 1900s on hours to be worked by student nurses. In 1911 the state had passed a law that women could not work more than 8 hours a day. However, the law did not cover student nurses, who worked much more than that. In 1912 a bill was introduced to include the students in the law. Doctors vigorously opposed the bill, with a Dr. Young stating that "the element of sacrifice is always present in true service." The superintendent of nurses in one hospital argued that schools of nursing would be hampered by instilling students with the principle of self-sacrifice if they had to adhere to the "self-centered eight hour law," and she asserted that real nursing could not be timed by the clock. Even the state nurses association passed a resolution opposing the bill. After the bill passed, nurses continued to deplore it; one superintendent of nurses wrote: "The eight hour law is still a heavy burden, really the most cruel thing they have ever done in the nursing profession. . . . Patients are complaining, head nurses work day and night doing the student nurses' work. . . . The eight hours has compelled us to increase the number of nurses three-fold, which also means more head nurses, maids, cooks, waiters, etc., etc." (Kalisch & Kalisch, 1975).

Skipping to my own student days, which began nearly half a century later, let me give you a glimpse of our typical schedule. After a very brief period of solely didactic instruction in the classroom (I think it was just a few months), we freshman students began a new schedule that included both clinical work and classes. Off we went to the floors to work "split shifts." I will tell you about split shifts because many of you are younger than I and escaped this ingenious way of scheduling student clinicals. The hours of work were perfectly timed to coincide with the hospital's needs for staffing. During the busy morning of breakfast, baths, procedures, and preparing patients for surgery, we students worked from 7:00 a.m. to 11:00 a.m.. Few of us really finished by 11:00, given an assignment of from 8 to 10 patients, so we hurriedly ate lunch in the cafeteria and ran down the hill to the nursing building for an afternoon of classes. Then back up the hill to the hospital we trudged to complete our 8 hours of clinical work, either from 3:00 p.m. to 7:00 p.m., which covered the return of patients from surgery, the frantic time of new admissions, and the evening meal, or from 7:00 p.m. to 11:00 p.m., which covered all of the evening treatments and procedures, administration of the backrubs, nourishments, and medications, and getting the patients settled down for the night before the night shift nurses came on duty. Of course, there was still studying to do, so there was no time remaining in the day for rest or recreation. We weren't allowed off the grounds for social outings, except on the weekends, anyway. On the weekends, we were often asked to "work extra" for pay, which many of us did because we really needed the money. The pressure to work these extra shifts was often intense, with appeals to our sense of compassion for the patients who needed care. I can remember being urged by a supervisor to cancel a date or other plans because the hospital badly needed someone to work on Saturday. My personal plans didn't matter; the hospital's needs were more important. I learned the concept of self-sacrifice well, and it is still with me.

I am not trying to denigrate my particular nursing school, because all of the diploma schools of the time were structured similarly. Nor am I trying to imply that I disliked nursing work, because that was not the case. I loved my work with the patients. I had—and still have—lots of energy, so that working long hours doesn't bother me. What I so acutely realize, however, is the superb job that was done by the faculty and the hospital administration to inculcate in me the belief that my own needs did not matter. From years of interacting with other nurses, I know that many of you learned the same lesson about sacrificing the self. For nurses who are women, the lesson was merely a reinforcement of our socialization to femininity. When we subsequently added roles as wives and mothers to our caregiving responsibilities, time for self-care was virtually extinguished. We began to feel like Eunice Adams, a participant in the Nurses Anger Study:

If I'm not pulled in that direction, I'm pulled in the other, and they're going to pull me apart one of these days. I just can't keep up with all their needs. I'm about tired. You do and you do and you do, and sometimes I think I'm just going to walk away and not come back.

A few years ago, there was an interesting study of married female nurses who had received a master's degree from Yale during the years 1941 to 1965. The tension between family and work commitments was examined in relation to the development of cardiovascular disease. Sacrifice was a key variable, both in terms of career limitations that women thought necessary because of family commitments and difficulty in relationships as a result of career involvement. Scoring high on sacrifice—trying to do everything for everybody—was found to be a significant predictor of major cardiovascular disease (Dixon, Dixon, & Spinner, 1991).

In a study of our own (Thomas & Donnellan, 1993), women's primary stressor was vicarious stress, the stress that results from taking on the burdens of other people. When we asked participants an open-ended question about their greatest stress, we expected to hear answers about their jobs or relationship dilemmas. But the number one category of responses pertained to events in the lives of others, such as their son's divorce, grandson's illness, unmarried daughter's pregnancy, nephew's car accident, eight-year-old's difficulties in school, aging parent's mental capacity, or daughter-in-law's mother's terminal illness. Such events are uncontrollable and therefore fuel a chronic impotent anger, because the individuals cannot "fix" things.

Sometimes women protect their husbands from stress by keeping news of such events from them. Social psychologist Ron Kessler, who interviewed husbands and wives separately for a stress study, was amazed at this tendency: "We would interview a woman and she would tell us her daughter had had an abortion. When we asked why her husband hadn't mentioned it, she would say, 'Oh, I didn't tell him' " (Kessler, cited in Turkington, 1985, p. 38). Carrying the husband's stress for him is clearly a remnant of women's gender role socialization to sacrifice the self in service to others. Carrying a lot of vicarious stress for their families and friends can be especially dangerous for nurses, who spend their work lives empathizing with others' pain. While I would never want nurses to cease being caring human beings, some detachment is necessary to avoid psychological overload.

The process of learning to achieve a balance between engagement and detachment in caregiving has been studied by Carmack (1997) in both formal caregivers (nurses, social workers, priests, etc.) and informal caregivers (friends or family of ill individuals). Almost all of the study participants had been overinvolved at some point and had suffered the consequences. They had learned through experience how to balance in order to survive. One study participant found it helpful to imagine a scale or seesaw. During the process of achieving a balance, caregivers became more realistic about their own inability to fix everything. They no longer took on the problems of the people they were helping, but instead allowed self-determination. They set limits and boundaries, such as refusing to work overtime or give their home phone numbers to patients. And all of them recognized the importance of practicing self-care.

I cannot emphasize strongly enough that it is time for us to care for ourselves. We must understand that honoring our own needs for rest and play not only is crucial for our health, but also enhances our capacity to give to others. Stressed, angry nurses who feel like running away from all the demands on them cannot be a healing presence to the patients they see. Therefore, self-care is not a "selfish" thing to do. It is likely that we will be even better nurses as a result.

A WORD TO WORKAHOLICS

Caring for the self begins by assessing both the work and the nonwork dimensions of your life. Could the word *workaholic* be used to describe you? If not, you can skip to the next section. Unfortunately, this noun applies not only to nurses but also to many other Americans who do professional work. Words come into our language when people have a need to name something. *Workaholic* is defined as "a person obsessively occupied with work at the expense of normal leisure, human relationships, etc." The key word, of course, is *obsessively*, when an individual's work behavior becomes like the obsessive drug-seeking behavior seen in addiction to chemicals. I have known some nurses whose entire life was nursing. At times, I have been close to deserving the workaholic label myself.

I, as a recovering workaholic, now know that work cannot be all of one's existence. Sociologist Arlie Hochschild, in her book *The Time Bind* (1997), draws some disturbing conclusions about workers who have an enormous investment of identity and self-worth in their jobs. They are spending increasing hours on the job and short-changing their families. Hochschild states, "Although work can complement—and indeed, improve—family life, in recent decades it has largely competed with family, and won" (Hochschild, 1997, cited in Bourke, 1997, p. 8B). Working parents drop their children off at day care in the wee hours of the morning and pick them up at the last possible moment at night. Dinner is fast food. Family rituals go by the wayside because no one has time. Work is the place where many people see their friends, reap rewards for performance, and escape the stresses of home. In contrast, home is the source of irritation and conflict. In effect, work has become home and home is work, according to Hochschild. It's a sobering analysis.

Victor Frankl survived horrendous treatment in a World War II concentration camp and went on to become a shrewd observer of postwar society. He knew that we were going astray when we began to put more emphasis on materialism than on the meaning of life: "For too long we have been dreaming a dream ... that if we just improve the socioeconomic situation of people, everything will be okay, people will become happy. The truth is that as the struggle for survival has subsided, the question has emerged: survival for what? Ever more people today have the means to live, but no meaning to live for" (Frankl, 1978, p. 21). Along the same vein, another giant of our times, Carl Jung, warned against preoccupation with the outward trappings of success while neglecting the inner life: "I have frequently seen people become neurotic when they content themselves with inadequate or wrong answers to the questions of life. They seek position, marriage, reputation, outward success or money, and remain unhappy and neurotic even when they have attained what they were seeking. Such people are usually confined within too narrow a spiritual horizon. Their life has not sufficient content, sufficient meaning" (Jung, 1965, p. 140). This may be a good time to take a moment to reflect on your purpose in life and your goals. Why are you doing what you're doing, and is it getting you what you want out of life?

REFLECTION ON YOUR PURPOSE IN LIFE AND GOALS

If we deprive ourselves of time for rest and contemplation, life can be like a speeding train, hurtling past forests, valleys, and rock formations, which we are too busy to appreciate. One day blends into another, weeks fold into months, and before you know it a whole year has whizzed by. We're not sure of the destination, but we are definitely being thrust forward toward something. I challenge you to step off the train for a bit. If you don't step off from time to time, physical illness or depression may bring you to a halt, especially if your itinerary needs some correction. I am concerned about nurses who seem to be unclear about where they are going. For example, Dawn Perkins, who was highly stressed and angry when interviewed for our research, is studying to be a nurse practitioner because her husband wants her to:

> *If you asked me what is my primary reason for going back to school, I'd tell you it's because my husband wants me to. Right now that's my only interest. I know that's not a good reason to do it, but when I start something, I finish it. I'm not going to quit. If I quit, I'd have less stress. [My husband is] putting a lot of pressure on me. He says things like, "Well, you can quit," but I know that he [doesn't] really mean that. I feel like if I make a B, he gets disappointed. I have no plans to know what I'll do as a [nurse practitioner]. I have no concept right now of what I want to do in that role.*

The great myths and religious traditions all contain sagas of heroes journeying to find their personal destinies. A Greek-derived word for fulfilling one's purpose in life is *entelechy*. I have heard psychologist Jean Houston say that it is the entelechy of an acorn to be an oak tree, and likewise the entelechy of each human to be uniquely who he or she is.

David Bohm might speak of the implicate order, Abraham Maslow of self-actualization, a Buddhist of karma. In some sense an inner force is creating and shaping us, but we are modifying it as well by the choices that we make. One of life's major choices, is, of course, our profession. But in today's turbulent times, this is not a choice made just once when we are in early adulthood. Professional directions must be renegotiated many times during a career. Many potentials of the self become evident only in middle or later adulthood. Many opportunities are not offered to us until we obtain additional experience or credentials.

Maslow, in describing self-actualizing people, said that work becomes a defining characteristic of the self, becomes part of the self. When you have found your niche, you are getting paid for doing what you love to do. Is this true of you at the present time? If it is not, what would excite and challenge you? Continuing to do work that is no longer engaging and satisfying is, to some extent, a death of the self (Levinson, 1996). One group of nurse authors claims that there are more nurses who are "bored out" than burned out (Simms, Erbin-Roesemann, Darga, & Coeling, 1990). In their study of 168 nurses, only 35 said they were very excited about their work. The researchers identified four factors that were significant predictors of work excitement. As you might expect, when frustration with (1) working conditions and (2) work arrangements was high, excitement was low. Positively related to work excitement were (3) variety in work experiences and (4) opportunity to grow and learn. Home care nurses had the highest level of excitement, differing significantly from nurses employed in critical care, general care, and rehabilitation, perhaps because of their greater autonomy. If your work has become routine or boring, maybe it's time to explore something different in an environment that fosters growth and learning. Do you have a plan for your career, or is it unfolding in a haphazard manner? Where do you want to be in your career 5 years from now? What would it take for you to get there? Do you need to go back to school? Do you need to pursue certification? What are your goals with regard to your relationships with family and friends? What would you like to be able to do in your leisure time? How could you build more pleasure into your harried existence?

BUILDING MORE PLEASURE INTO YOUR LIFE

Barasch (1993) has pointed out that the "workweek" of our tribal ancestors was about 20 hours; the remainder of their time was spent in conversation and play (singing, dancing, etc.). It's ironic that we, their sophisticated descendants, with our self-cleaning ovens and store-bought bread, can't find the time for play. We do have conversation, with our e-mail and voice mail and cell phones, but not long, deep dialogue before a great fire, talking far into the night as the flames grow low and the embers turn to ash. Deep conversation can be highly pleasurable, filling our need for meaningful connections with others.

One of the best stress-busters after a grueling workday is distraction. Take off your uniform—or your dress-for-success business suit—and slip into the happy hedonism of Jimmy Buffett. Make a margarita, non-alcoholic if you choose, and put some shrimp on to boil. Let the music take you to the Caribbean, where the sun bakes everyone into a slowed-down lethargy and your only decision is when to turn over and let the sun warm your other side. Or perhaps you'd rather go to San Francisco, where you left your heart, or New Orleans, where the saints go marching in. Music can take you there, for a delightful mini-vacation.

Even when you're still steaming from an unpleasant confrontation just before you left work, the research of Zillman (1988) suggests that your anger can be diminished or terminated by highly absorbing, pleasant entertainment. A movie can quickly transport you to the breathtaking vistas of Alaska or the Alps, or to the vast desert or the canyons of the American West. Caught up in the visual images and the story, it becomes impossible for you to continue to dwell on your problems. Dance performances, plays, concerts, and poetry readings await you in any area. Even small towns have theater troupes and choral groups. I hesitate to recommend television, because I think that most Americans spend too much of their free time in front of their TV sets, in a kind of bland, anesthetized stupor, but TV may be pleasurable to you. If so, pop the popcorn and plop down in front of the set.

I can hear some of you—especially women—saying that these recreational activities sound great, but how will the housecleaning and laundry get done? One of women's biggest dissatisfactions in the Women's Anger Study (Thomas, 1993b; Thomas et al., in press) was the failure of their partners to take a fair share of the household chores. This segment of a phenomenological interview is illustrative:

> *I felt like my weekends were spent cleaning the house while [my husband's] weekends were spent playing, and I resented that. . . . Like I told him when I was angry, "You don't want to compare what you do and what I do because you'll lose; trust me. How many times do you do the laundry, and how many times do you fold and put up clothes, and cook the meals and*

run the kids?" He knows he doesn't do that. He knows I do most of it, and he likes it that way and he wants to keep it that way.

I have found that when wives in my anger workshops make a specific assertive request, most husbands are willing to help out. Instead, many women are fuming about the inequitable division of labor in silence, expecting their husbands to intuit that they need assistance. This is an irrational expectation. Link your assertive request to an outcome that will be pleasurable for both of you: "If we finish the chores by 11:00, there's still time to get to the mountains for a picnic." Try it.

HUMOR

Yes, I know. There are days when the only way you can put a smile on your face is by putting a coat hanger in your mouth. But if that's what it takes, do it. Humor is inexpensive, widely available, and it can be self-administered. It's even better when it's shared with other nurses. Laughing with one another alleviates the seriousness that permeates our work settings and counters our sense of isolation, providing important moments of genuine connection. You can probably gauge the emotional health of a work group by the amount of laughter members share: People are most likely to be humorous and playful in the presence of others who like and enjoy them (Saussy, 1995).

Humor can be used to dispel anger at a provocation. A few years ago, when the first reports of our research on women's anger hit the press, I was inundated with calls from reporters. Most of the journalists were responsible individuals who read at least some of the book before conducting their interviews, asked me intelligent questions, and preparing stories that were reasonably accurate. Some of the journalists, such as Jane Brody of the *New York Times,* did a superb job describing the study and its findings. Not so Rush Limbaugh. Without interviewing me or taking any other steps to verify the accuracy of his story, he went on the radio and trashed the research. The first I knew of Rush's diatribe was about 15 minutes after his show went off the air. A professor from the College of Education had heard the broadcast while driving to the university and, outraged on my behalf, came straight to my office in the College of Nursing to tell me about it. My first response was anger, but then I considered the source and became amused. By the time other friends were calling to express their dismay about the unfair comments,

I was laughing and saying that I planned to add "trashed by Rush Limbaugh" to my vita.

TEARS

Tears get a bad rap in our society. They are acceptable only in young children and only until a certain age, after which they are disparaged. No one wants to be called a crybaby. Although in adulthood tears are somewhat more permissible for women than for men, women who freely cry still run the risk of being labeled overly emotional or hysterical. Crying for men receives even more pejorative labeling. You may recall that public crying actually crushed the presidential aspirations of Edmund Muskie. My husband grew up in a Mediterranean culture, and he finds Americans far too uptight about crying. It's not unusual for him, and other men from his part of the world, to cry.

I believe that crying can be therapeutic, releasing emotional tension and leaving in its place a cleansed, quiet state. The only major study on crying in adults (Frey & Langseth, 1985) was devoted to a chemical analysis of tears and their physiological function. I found the study results interesting, however. Emotional tears were chemically different from irritant tears (e.g., caused by those pollutants) in that they serve an excreting function. Analysis showed that emotional tears contain chemicals that may mediate the immune system's response to stress. This research raises an intriguing question: By stifling our tears, are we depriving ourselves of a natural healing mechanism that could combat the ill effects of angry, stressful situations? I say that having a good cry at the end of a frustrating workday is a healthy way of caring for oneself. Go ahead and let those tears flow.

EXERCISE

You already know that you need to be exercising. Studies show that exercise lifts your spirits for as long as 2 to 4 hours (Kaplan, 1997). But did you also know that the greatest improvements in emotional state occur when people feel worst before they engage in exercise (Gauvin, Rejeski, & Norris, 1996)? Given these demonstrated benefits for droopy spirits, coupled with what you already know about heart health, muscle tone, and so on, what's getting in your way of exercising? A common excuse I hear from nurses about their failure to exercise is "no time to get to the health club." I always chuckle a bit, wondering how so many of us have gotten the idea that fitness can only be achieved if one has a health club membership—or a personal trainer. True enough, health clubs offer all those snazzy rowing machines, treadmills, weight contraptions, and other devices to make you puff, sweat, and groan. But what would our parents' generation think about trotting off to the health club instead of just attacking some chores at home? After a day of hoeing and milking and chopping cotton, I doubt if any of my rural West Tennessee relatives ever had to worry about fitness.

Those of us who are suburban couch sitters do. Although I sped down the hospital halls in my "duty shoes" with the best of them when I was younger, my current work at the university is largely sedentary. My colleagues who are therapists, middle managers, and administrators spend much of their day sitting as well. And even nurses whose work is entirely in fast-paced settings such as emergency departments or intensive care units cannot count on getting enough aerobic exercise during the workday. Remember that for aerobic benefit, your heart rate must be raised to within 50% to 70% of its maximum (for a man, that is 220 beats per minute minus his age; for a woman, 200 minus her age).

Many people are turned off by intensely competitive sports. The good news is that you need not take up racquetball to be fit. It's relatively easy to build many health-promoting activities into your daily routine. I think the best way to begin is by shelving all those labor-saving devices in the kitchen and the garage and start burning calories doing work the way we used to do. Why in the world do we think we need to have riding mowers to take care of postage stamp–sized lawns? Why do we need to pay somebody else an exorbitant amount to wash and vacuum the car? Writer Harry Chipkin in an article in "Family Health" provided a list of such activities and the amount of calories they burn, as compared with calories expended in vigorous sports like squash. According to Chipkin's Sports-haters, Nonathletic, Easy-does-it, Kiss-your-sweatsuit-goodbye Equivalency Rating, or SNEAKER, washing the car for an hour is equivalent to swimming for an hour, and mowing the lawn with a manual mower for 75 minutes is roughly the same as playing racquetball for 35 minutes. Ironing for 3 hours is about the same as cross-country skiing for 30 minutes, and heavy scrubbing burns 250 to 350 calories per hour. One of my favorite facts is that climbing stairs burns 250% more calories than swimming for the same amount of time, 150% more than tennis, 94% more than racquetball, 63% more than cycling, and 23% more than running. You really don't have to jog down the boulevard, pounding the asphalt while breathing in all that carbon monoxide. Instead, you can run up and down the stairs in the comfort of your own home.

You may be thinking that ironing and scrubbing are extremely unappealing ways to get your exercise. Whether or not any of Chipkin's ideas appeal to you, resolve to get your body moving. Fitness does not mean just cardiac improvement but also greater flexibility, endurance, and strength, improvements in metabolism of sugar and lipids, and decreased tension and stress. The latter benefit is particularly important during times of emotional turmoil at work. Research shows that biking at a moderate rate for an hour reduces depression, anger, and confusion. However, the same research shows that moderation is the key. When individuals who were upset cycled more intensely or strained to their absolute limit, they actually felt worse afterward (Motl, cited in Kaplan, 1997).

I find the tendency to push oneself to exhaustion a uniquely American phenomenon. We exercise like we work: in obsessive Type A fashion. Nowhere else in the world have I seen so many grim-faced, driven runners. Examples of a healthier approach to body movement abound in other cultures. One of the fondest memories of my 1985 visit to China was the sight of thousands of people outdoors in the early morning doing their exercises, graceful octogenarians included. Even in the hospitals that I visited, all patients who could be ambulatory were exercising, out on the roof garden in the fresh air wherever possible. In China, movement is considered as important for health as eating and sleeping. We can learn from other cultures.

Perhaps one secret of the Chinese dedication to exercise is the communal nature of the activity. People do tai chi movements together in public parks and other community gathering places. In our country, many of us are more likely to engage in physical activity if we are enrolled in a class or have a neighbor to jog with. Owning a dog provides the impetus for some people to be active. Writer Carol Krucoff (1997) points out that dogs are excuse-proof, need no batteries or electricity, and are impossible to ignore when they want to go out for their morning jaunt. She has learned some "health secrets" from exercising with her beagle: (1) Greet everyone you meet, but keep your ears cocked until you determine friend or foe; (2) lap up water every chance you get; (3) enjoy nature in all its moods; (4) stretch frequently; (5) live in the moment; (6) rely on more than just your sense of sight; (7) always take time to roll on the floor and play; and (8) never become too busy to stop and smell the rabbit holes. Terrific advice, in my opinion! Get off the couch—with or without a dog—and go move your body. You'll live longer, look better, feel great, and be an excellent example for your patients.

MEDITATION

Another useful self-care strategy is the practice of meditation. Meditation has many documented benefits, including the reduction of stress levels (Tsai & Crockett, 1993). When I talk about this practice to my students, some of them raise the objection that it is connected with certain religions such as Buddhism. Because many of my students are Southern Baptists, they think that meditation is inappropriate for them to do. I try to give them readings containing accurate information, but the decision to meditate is, of course, ultimately theirs.

What is meditation, and why are some individuals leery of it? "Meditation refers to a family of techniques which have in common a conscious attempt to focus attention in a nonanalytical way and an attempt not to dwell on discursive, ruminating thought" (Shapiro, 1982, p. 268). I suppose some people are leery of it because of its unfair association with misguided individuals in the '60s who dropped out to wander aimlessly on the fringes of society.

Breathing meditation is perhaps least likely to provoke objections on the grounds of religion, because concentration on breathing is a part not only of Buddhist and Hindu practices, but also of Judeo-Christian traditions. Kornfield (1993) says that the breath is a great teacher, from whom we can learn about opening and letting go. His recommended procedure for breathing meditation is as follows: To begin, find a quiet place to sit. Select a regular time in the morning or evening. If you like, read something inspirational. Then begin your period of meditation. Bring your attention to your breathing. Let your breath change rhythms naturally. When your mind wanders, simply come back to the next breath. When you return, acknowledge where you wandered with a soft word: *thinking* or *planning*. At first, keep your sessions to 10 to 20 minutes.

Meditation is very much like training a puppy, according to Kornfield: Imagine a playful puppy you have told to "stay," but the puppy scampers off in a flash. Again, you sit the puppy down and say, "Stay," but the puppy continues to run away. Likewise, in training yourself to meditate, be prepared for an unruly mind that just will not stay focused. Infinite patience will be required before you end up with the puppy as your lifelong friend. But you will gradually learn to calm and center yourself using breath meditation.

Walking meditation is a variant that I find appealing. It involves selecting a place where you can quietly walk back and forth, indoors or out, about 10 to 30 paces. Begin by closing your eyes and centering yourself, feeling your body. Then open your eyes and begin to walk slowly, easily, paying attention as you place each foot. When you reach the end of your path, pause, carefully turn, and start back. Walk for 10 to 20 minutes. When the mind wanders, follow the same procedure as above. After you have some practice with walking meditation, you can do it informally when walking down a street or to and from your car. It is a simple but profoundly different way of walking than you usually do when your mind is preoccupied with thinking and planning (Kornfield, 1993).

IMMERSING OURSELVES IN THE SACRED

Caring for the self also involves taking time to immerse yourself in whatever you find sacred. Doing what is sacred to you is not necessarily what your parents, or theologians, or society may consider sacred; the sacred is that which has the power to move you deeply and help you cope with the demands and struggles of life's journey. You may find the sacred in music, poetry, art, or gardening (Muff, 1995). Alice Walker calls her writing a prayer. Many Americans are hungry for new ways to care for the soul, as shown by the popularity of the books by Thomas Moore on this topic.

Being in nature is incredibly important to me. I find a cathedral of trees more awe-inspiring than a manmade one, a rainbow more spectacular than a stained glass window. I live in a beautiful part of the world, with gently curving hills, so lovely in the spring with new vegetation softening their creases, smoothing out the corrugated evidence of erosion. Taking a drive, I am immersed in a vast sea of green fields and blue-gray hills. Ride along with me and see the wispy, tentative, fragile green of willow wands waving in the breeze . . . a richer yellow-green vista in the background, the texture of velvet, like a pillow cover tightly stretched over a fat, round cushion of soil . . . the darker green of spiky pines punctuating all this softness and roundness . . . a flamboyant forsythia thrusting itself into my line of vision, Bradford pear trees in their lacy bridal white, pearly gray rock families clustered like mushrooms on the hillsides, a random daffodil here and there . . . in the sky, ephemeral cloud curls suffused with pink-rose of early morning sun . . . the clouds patterning and repatterning: now a herd of droll, woolly sheep, now a nest of elegant white birds with primly folded feathers, now frothy peaks of meringue . . . the sun becoming more brilliant in a sky that is the color of Lake Louise . . . the hills light-dappled, serene, solid, wise, eternal. Hear the hum of the universe and the heartbeat of God.

IV

Claiming Our Power

10

Taking a New Stance Toward the Concept of Power

> Personal power is a flame within me that I have to follow
> to be me. It looks like a tiny flame that could be easily
> blown out but really it's one of those perpetual lights.
> I can go off and leave it or give some of it to others
> and feel confident that it won't go out. In fact, the
> more I give my flame to others, the brighter my flame
> gets, until I don't have to worry about its going out at
> all. It comes from inside of me but it's brightened by
> others so that I can proudly say, "Look, this is my
> flame" and I can follow it. All of my important life
> decisions are made by the light of this flame. It's the
> light of integrity, of being true to myself.
>
> Stratman, 1990, p. 5896B

For a long time now I have been using the word *empowerment* in my speeches and workshops. The term is used in different ways in the more than 400 papers on the topic that have been published within the past 12 years. Let me explain what I mean by it. I define *empowerment* as the enhanced ability to take action and resolve problems. Empowerment theory and praxis have roots in feminist scholarship, adult education techniques, and community and political organization methods (Gutierrez, 1990). Self-empowerment, which this book is designed to facilitate, means having the power to influence and control one's own life (Heide,

1988). But beyond controlling their own lives, nurses must become empowered to make a greater impact on institutional and health care policies. Too many nurses remain marginalized or silenced, chafing at shortsighted policies but excluded from the decision-making circle. Davies (1995) maintains that nurses are usually excluded from policy debates because they are considered "incompetent" or "divided." When they do enter the arena of debate, they often feel "bruised and confused."

I contend that anger can be empowering, if it is used constructively. It is when we get angry that we are moved to act. Strong emotion galvanizes us to challenge sex discrimination, harassment, inequitable work assignments, and ill-conceived policies (Thomas & Droppleman, 1997). We need look no further than the founder of modern nursing for corroboration of my premise. Recall that Florence Nightingale said, "I do well to be angry" (Strachey, 1996, p. 31). It was Nightingale's chafing at the uselessness of the Victorian lady's social role that fueled her resolve to "strive after a better life for women" (Cook, 1913, p. 102). It was her outrage at the deplorable sanitation, nutrition, and medical care of the British soldiers that brought about massive reforms, not only in the Crimea but also back home in England. It was her passionate commitment to education for nurses that brought modern professional nursing into existence. It was her righteous anger that propelled her into the public policy arena to address prostitution, crime, infant mortality, workhouse conditions, and the problems of the rural poor.

The power of the written word was her forte, and her tactics are still worthy of emulation today. For example, Nightingale often wrote to the same individual numerous times until the desired action had been completed. She also used the technique of repetition of key points within the body of a letter (Monteiro, 1985). In addition to her persuasive letters (at least 15,000 of which have been found), she published 147 books and pamphlets and submitted numerous reports to Queen Victoria, Parliament, government commissions, and newspapers. Many of these documents included skillfully prepared graphs, charts, tables, and figures based on statistics she had gathered to bolster her arguments.

Clearly, Nightingale had "fire in the belly" for her causes and used it to great effect. Likewise, I think that anger can ignite the "fire" that contemporary nurses need for bold actions at this critical time. It can propel us into the societal debates regarding who should get what health care services, from whom, and where.

It is a truism that no one gives away power. Nurses themselves are going to have to make an effort to take it. But nursing is ambivalent toward the concept of power, perhaps because it has remained a woman's profession (Garant, 1981). As Levinson (1996) found in his sample of career women, authority is equated with authoritarianism—the unilateral, exploitive use of power. Thus, the women could not acknowledge, even to themselves, that they wanted positions of authority and power. Nightingale was an unusual woman who defied Victorian society's rules for her gender, but few of the nurse leaders who followed her displayed similar courage. Many women in nursing today view power as something unfeminine or coercive (Carlson-Catalano, 1994). At one conference I attended, Pat Schroeder, the former member of Congress, exhorted women to unbind our minds, alleging that our minds have been bound just as the feet of Chinese women once were bound. Statistics support the truth of Schroeder's allegation for nurses: In a study by Valentine (1992) five out of six nurses regarded power and ambition negatively. Nurses who fought for their rights were viewed as uncaring and undeserving, "not having the qualities that nurses should have" (p. 20). Presumably, those qualities that nurses should have were humility, self-sacrifice, and bearing one's burden in silence. Not long ago, I was fascinated to learn that the motto chosen for the first school of nursing in Canada, St. Catharine's, was "I see but I am silent" (George, 1997). How accurately this motto captures the traditional role socialization of the student nurse! We recited the Nightingale pledge, but we sure weren't encouraged to behave like Nightingale. Instead of learning to be persuasive and powerful when we were in school, we learned to keep our mouths shut and do as we were told, lest we be labeled "troublemakers."

The sense of powerlessness that permeated our nurse interview data was one of the most disturbing aspects of the research. Powerlessness was identified in earlier studies of nurses too. Bush (1988) found that powerlessness was a major cause of job dissatisfaction in hospital nurses. Erlen and Frost (1991) had set out to study nurses' experience in influencing ethical decisions. However, what they found was pervasive powerlessness described by nurses of all ages, educational levels, and years of nursing experience. Nurses were unable to effect resolution to situations, resulting in anger, frustration, and exhaustion. As in our own study, the nurses had knowledge and responsibility but lacked the corresponding authority.

I know you've heard the maxim about power corrupting. Heide (1988) proposed a corollary: that powerlessness corrupts and absolute powerlessness corrupts absolutely. The "corruption" takes many forms, including decreased self-confidence, inhibited personal and professional growth, competition with other powerless nurses for a modicum of power, and identification with the powerful oppressor, as we discussed in Chapter 5. When a group has been powerless for a long time, its members come to believe that "this is the way things are."

POWER: WE HAVE TO WANT IT BEFORE WE CAN HAVE IT

It's time for nurses to take a new stance toward the concept of power. We need to claim our power. Power may be as fundamental to human existence as anxiety, self-concept, and self-esteem (Pieranunzi, 1997). In her book *Paths to Power,* Natasha Josefowitz (1980) distinguishes between power as forcefulness and power as effectiveness. It is effective power that I advocate: power that enables us to make positive, proactive changes. We have to want it before we can have it. We have to believe that there is enough of it to go around so that we can stop hoarding our thimblefuls of it. We have to understand that you can build power by building relationships with colleagues and by pooling talents and resources. When each of us as individuals becomes empowered, the power quotient of the group increases; likewise, the group's power can enhance the development and functioning of its individual members. Power is a network of practices carried out by many people. There is creativity in power, as shown in a study of African tribal societies. Rejecting conceptions of power as subjugation and domination, these tribal societies see power as a means to "create new forms of experience and activity" (Arens & Karp, cited in Pieranunzi, 1997, p. 161). Surely there has never been a more critical time for the nursing society to create new forms of activity.

The empowerment process involves four interrelated psychological changes that take place, not necessarily in a precise sequence. First, developing a personal sense of self-efficacy or mastery is essential in moving from apathy to action. Second, it is necessary to develop a group consciousness, meaning a keen awareness of the shared powerlessness of nurses and the factors that have created it. Third, we must be clear that there is no need for self-blame because we are not responsible for the inequitable power arrangements in our work settings that have long oppressed us. Finally, each of us must assume personal responsibility for change (Gutierrez, 1990).

WHAT NURSE ADMINISTRATORS CAN DO

The nurse administrator can play a number of vital roles in empowering staff: model, mentor, challenger, facilitator, problem-solver, supporter. It does not diminish one's power to lift others on the climb up the ladder. To the extent that autonomy of staff can be increased through decentralization, self-scheduling, and other innovations, the anger "titer" of the institution will decrease.

A number of new unit-level governance structures are being tried, and evaluation data about their impact on staff nurse job satisfaction is beginning to appear in the literature (Hastings & Waltz, 1995). The data indicate that some nurse managers have difficulty letting go and allowing their staff to participate in decision-making. However, involvement in decision-making is one of the strongest predictors of staff nurse job satisfaction. In participative management strategies, individuals throughout the organization are given more information and power. The result? A true win-win situation. Not only do the staff appreciate the freedom to make decisions, but studies show that the managers who work in decentralized hospitals have higher job satisfaction (Acorn, Ratner, & Crawford, 1997). Likewise, nursing faculty members have greater job satisfaction in institutions where there is less formalization and centralization (Mansen, 1993).

Fostering staff intrapreneurship is one proven way of empowering staff. Intrapreneurs have creative ideas and implement them within their place of employment instead of establishing a separate business, as entrepreneurs do. For example, intrapreneurs at 3M developed those indispensable yellow Post-it notes. In a pilot program at the University of Michigan Hospitals, proposals from nursing service personnel are solicited for new products, processes, or programs and then evaluated by a senior management team. When a proposal is selected for further development, the intrapreneur is matched with a mentor-coach to prepare a business plan. Innovators are honored at a reception given by the hospital CEO. Nurses have responded with excitement and enthusiasm to this program (Marszalek-Gaucher & Elsenhans, 1988).

There are several other published success stories about intrapreneurship. Boyar and Martinson (1990) advocate an Intrapreneurial Group Practice Model, which has been implemented in several locales. In one hospital in Albuquerque, nursing staff prepared a proposal, made budget decisions, and drew up marketing plans. Middle management was completely eliminated, and work groups of staff nurses now make all day-to-day management decisions, reporting directly to a patient care director (Davidson, 1987). At Johns Hopkins in Baltimore, groups of nurses were empowered to make their own case assignments. The groups are overseen by committees that deal with scheduling, education, peer review, and quality assurance. The staff nurses receive a quarterly bonus based on their unit's productivity. Documented benefits for the institution include decreases in staff sick time and turnover (York & Fecteau, 1987). These reports show what can happen when management gives nurses permission and support to run with their ideas.

In a 3-year study that evaluated the outcome of training activities to increase nurses' power in practice settings, Gorman and Clark (1986) found administrative support to be a crucial element. The reseachers assigned 170 nurses from nine metropolitan hospitals to either an experimental group (which participated in the training activities) or a control group (which went about their usual nursing practice activities). Nurses in the experimental group were taught to apply their analytic skills to organizational problems, to work in teams on planned change projects, to use their colleagues for consultation and support, and to function in a complex bureaucracy. The directors of nursing services in the nine hospitals played key roles in the project. They provided access to resources, information, and support systems, and they interacted with the staff nurses as professional colleagues. Many of the nurses had had no previous contact with nursing leadership, even when they had worked for their institutions for an extended period of time. Findings of the study showed that members of the experimental group scored higher on outcome measures of nursing power. This successful and worthwhile project could be replicated in other settings by enlightened nurse administrators who understand Kanter's contention that *"when more people are empowered—that is, allowed to have control over the conditions that make their actions possible—then more is accomplished, more gets done"* (Kanter, 1977, p. 166).

WHAT YOU CAN DO TO ENHANCE THE POWERFUL SELF

1. Engage in a power analysis. If you are a researcher, you have learned an entirely different meaning for this term, but here I am using power analysis to mean identifying potential sources of power in your present work situation. When you have completed your analysis, set some specific goals to work toward. Knowledge is power. You already have highly specialized clinical knowledge or

you could not be functioning as a nurse in today's world. But you probably need to learn more about business and health policy. Did you know that Tom Peters, in his book *Thriving on Chaos* (1987), estimated that the average staff nurse manages $2 million in business each day? Acquiring knowledge about trending, budgeting, marketing, and cost-benefit analysis—topics that I bet you didn't cover in nursing school—will give you an advantage when promotions are considered. Make sure that others are aware of your special knowledge or expertise.

Find out where decisions are made and try to get yourself appointed or elected to a spot on the committee or board that decides. Once appointed, show up for meetings. You don't have any power if you aren't there. Bring data with you to the meetings to document your arguments. If you've got the facts and figures, it's hard for an opponent to discount your proposal. When asked to assume a new responsibility, run with the opportunity instead of shrinking from it. Do a good job, because people will remember. Work on remembering names, analyzing group dynamics, and cultivating a network of influential contacts. Update forgotten skills and acquire new ones (computer skills are an extremely marketable commodity right now). Build a unique repertoire of talents. Make yourself indispensable to your work unit and your institution. One successful woman at our university recommends periodically asking, "If I leave the job tomorrow, will the show go on without a hitch? If the answer is yes, then I haven't positioned myself well." Good advice!

2. Take an assertiveness class. Assertiveness is defined as "behavior which enables a person to act in his own best interests, to stand up for himself without undue anxiety, to express his honest feelings comfortably, or to exercise his own rights without denying the rights of others" (Alberti & Emmons, 1974, p. 2). Assertive behavior is aimed at equalizing the balance of power, not putting down another person. A basic assertive statement when you are angry is a firm, clear statement ("I am angry") followed by the reason "because _____," then a request for what you would like to be different. The "broken record" technique can be used to calmly repeat the message several times if the other person doesn't seem to get it. Try this technique if someone is tuning you out or yelling while you speak.

When delivering an assertive message, lean forward confidently, keep direct eye contact, and don't hesitate, plead, or apologize.

Keep your message short, rather than cluttering it with excess information that will not be necessary to get the point across. No-no's while making your statement are a hostile, sarcastic tone, accusations, or blaming the other person for your angry feeling. Assertiveness is a skill that must be practiced. I highly recommend a class that involves role playing and feedback. Classes are frequently offered by university counseling centers and mental health facilities. If you are a faculty member, consider conducting a class for your nursing students after you are comfortable with your own skills. Some years ago, I developed an 11-week plan and conducted the assertiveness training sessions concurrently with the psychiatric-mental health nursing course I taught (Thomas, 1982). Assertiveness instruction would also be valuable in leadership and management courses.

3. Make your "bubble" bigger. Your assertive words will have greater impact if they are accompanied by assertive body language. I have used an exercise called "Making Your Bubble Bigger" with students for years. I got the idea from the "First Venusian Anthropological Expedition to Earth" by Nancy Henley. In Henley's (1977) story, Venusians visiting Earth observe that "all Earthlings have a space bubble around them, the amount of space belonging to their own bodies. Dominants have larger space bubbles. . . . One need only watch the Earthlings move about in their bubbles of different sizes, approaching bubble to bubble, to know immediately who is the superior, and who the inferior, in any interaction." (p. 27). You can watch the powerful "earthlings"—CEO's, doctors, lawyers—and see for yourself how big their bubbles are. You can make your bubble bigger too.

First, pick a private time and place where you can concentrate, uninterrupted, on expanding your bubble. Stretch out from the tips of your toes up through the top of your head. Stand tall and straight; make huge, expansive arm and hand gestures; walk around the room like you're royalty. Feel your bubble growing bigger, taking up more space. Sense the increased power and self-confidence that you have as a regal leader. If you like, practice in front of a mirror, paying particular attention to your posture, effective hand gestures, and walking with a determined gait. Then try out your new body language in a low-risk situation, (e.g., with a store clerk or waiter who's ignoring you). Later, try making your bubble bigger in increasingly complex situations.

4. Never acquiesce to the status quo when you are in a frustrating work situation in which you feel powerless. Unfortunately, women are more likely to do so than men. Mainiero (1986) talked to men and women about work situations of powerlessness and found a much higher percentage of women responding by acquiescence. That is, they acted in a helpless, dependent manner, like the nurses in our sample who had avowed that there was nothing they could do. In contrast, men were more likely to adopt a strategy of persuasion, discussing the frustrating situation persistently with the person who could supply a remedy. My motto is "Doing something always feels better than doing nothing." I am enough of a realist to know that none of us will ever achieve a work situation that is perfect. But you will feel better that you acted on your concerns.

5. Master the art of persuasion. You cannot acquire or exert power unless you are verbally articulate. Classes in speech-making or debate techniques can be helpful in learning how to mount an argument and deliver it with maximum impact. Such classes frequently involve videotaping so that you can see yourself as others see you. Classmates can be helpful in critiquing your hand gestures and other distracting mannerisms that detract from your overall effectiveness. Linguist Deborah Tannen (1994) points out that *how* you deliver your message is of crucial importance. Don't preface your remarks with disclaimers such as "I don't know if this will work, but . . ." or "You may have already tried this, but . . ." Speak with certainty and repeat key points. This way of speaking is more difficult for women, who tend to lower their voices, hesitate, and make disclaimers when arguing a position (Tannen, 1994).

Take your powers of persuasion out into the world. Join your district nurses association and community groups, taking the microphone to practice your skills in speaking to a main motion or defending a position. My district nurses association was definitely a leadership training ground for me over the years. People who know me now do not believe this, but I used to be very hesitant to speak before a group. When I first attended a state convention as a delegate, in 1965, I was nervous about just going to the podium at the district meeting afterward to give my delegate's report. Who would have dreamed that someday I would be on "Good Morning America" and making speeches to hundreds at ANA meetings? But as I became more involved in organizational work, I became much more comfortable in speaking, proposing actions, persuading others to support a plan I had concocted, debating without being overly emotional, convening caucuses to negotiate compromises, and other vital skills. I watched ANA leaders who had these skills and tried to emulate them. Persuasive speakers like Barbara Nichols, Gretta Styles, Luther Christman, Lucille Joel, Ginna Betts, and Bev Malone were my role models. I thank them for providing examples of the positive uses of power.

How will we know when we have achieved personal empowerment? According to psychologist Judith Worell (1996), an empowered individual has these characteristics:

Positive self-esteem, self-valuing
Positive comfort-distress quotient
Internal personal control
Avoidance of self-deprecation
Flexibility in gendered beliefs and behaviors
Assertiveness
Knowledge of important resources

These characteristics should look rather familiar to you, as much of the content of this book has been devoted to recommended actions to improve your self-esteem, lessen distress, and enhance control and assertiveness. But we're not quite finished. Worell says—and I heartily agree—that an empowered individual also has competence in problem-solving and acts as a change agent and social activist. Empowerment is an empty concept unless linked to a commitment to challenging oppression (Ward & Mullender, 1991). Once empowered, nurses must use their intelligence, creativity, and political savvy to address the problems in the profession. Read on to find out more about the process of problem-solving.

11

Solving Problems

> We are all faced with a series of great opportunities—
> brilliantly disguised as unsolvable problems.
>
> John Gardner

There are three kinds of people: those who make things happen, those who watch things happen, and those who don't know what's happening. This chapter is for those of you who want to make things happen, to solve the problems that interfere with your ability to practice your profession in the way that you want. Although much of our research data focused on unhealthy anger, some nurses used their anger productively. For example, Linda Harvey, a med-surg nurse, was able to advocate for herself when she alone was charged with a medication error for which at least one other person should have been held responsible. She explained to the director of nursing that although she was in error when she administered potassium to a patient who'd been taken off the supplement, the outgoing nurse hadn't flagged the change in orders in the Kardex or the chart and had forgotten to tell Linda about it at shift report. The hospital's medication error report form was subsequently revised to accommodate shared responsibility, and hospital policy was modified to put more red flags into effect when changes were made to a patient's medication regimen. Because of Linda's actions, nurses who make a medication error at that hospital now experience a less punitive aftermath.

Let's look at some of the other problems that nurses told us about and what can be done to solve them. Stressful, emotionally upsetting events come with the territory in nursing. But research shows that problem-focused coping is significantly correlated with a reduction in psychological stress symptoms (Hedin, 1994). As Pat Schroeder put it, "You

can't roll up your sleeves and wring your hands at the same time." Later
in the chapter, a number of nursing leaders candidly share their experiences of rolling up their sleeves and grappling with some tough situations. As you read their stories, keep the following principles in mind.

PRINCIPLES OF PROBLEM-SOLVING

Bedell and Lennox (1996) have proposed seven guiding principles of
problem-solving:

1. Learn to view problems as a natural part of life. It is not bad to
   have problems, nor does their presence imply weakness.
2. Think before jumping to a solution. It is more adaptive to do some
   thinking about the problem before attempting to solve it.
3. Engage in the process of problem-solving with the conviction that
   most problems can be solved.
4. Take responsibility for problems that can be attributed (at least in
   part) to yourself.
5. State what you can do, not what you can't do. Having a goal provides direction and incentive.
6. Consider whether your solution to the problem is legally and socially acceptable.
7. Consider whether your solution to the problem is within your
   power and ability. The most common error people make when
   problem-solving is forgetting that they can control only their own
   behavior.

IF YOU'RE BEATEN DOWN BY BUREAUCRACY

A host of studies show that it is not nursing work that causes nurses to
burn out, but the impediments to self-determined practice. The restrictions of bureaucratic institutions stifle nurses' creativity and independence. The following is an example of transforming a workplace. As the
nurses themselves described their situation, they were part of a "fiercely
patriarchal and autocratic hospital culture" (Breda et al., 1997, p. 77).
Fortunately, they understood that if changes were to occur, their own
actions would have to be the catalyst. So a small group of psychiatric
nurses at this New England hospital undertook a project to increase the
autonomy of nurses there. The project involved a number of elements,
including formation of a study group to prepare for certification, incor-

poration of new holistic healing interventions into their nursing practice, presentation of educational sessions and retreats for the staff, and increased participation in multidisciplinary teams. From an oppressed group, the nurses evolved to become increasingly confident, outspoken, and articulate:

> *The . . . project allowed us to experience a new sense of dignity about ourselves as professionals, which we call "ownership of practice." Ownership of practice includes many of the dimensions of autonomy—control over our practice, the freedom to make decisions, and the quality of professional exchange with colleagues that we always sought. We also [became] mentors and role models for less experienced and new nurses. Above all, we developed a firm sense of making a difference with clients and within the organization as a whole. We had become secure in our knowledge base and were no longer willing to be subordinated by others. We recognized that autonomy is linked to power and that the many limits placed on our practice were simply a way to keep nurses in line. (Breda et al., 1997, p. 79)*

The story has a happy ending. Physicians and social workers responded positively to the newly empowered nurses. In fact, the only resistance they encountered was from a few nurses who did not want to become more autonomous. These nurses had been well indoctrinated to believe that "the hospital knows what's best for us," and they saw no benefit of change. This successful project shows that nurses can challenge institutional rules and norms that limit their autonomy. Instead of leaving for better conditions, like so many nurses opt to do, Breda and her colleagues stayed in the same system and transformed it.

IF YOU'RE BEING SEXUALLY HARASSED

As shown in our research data, both male and female nurses are sexually harassed, despite greater societal consciousness-raising about harassment. Nurses will continue to be harassed until more of us take action to report—and prevent—its occurrence. Even though there have been some highly publicized lawsuits in recent years, statistics show that 90% of episodes of harassment in this country are not reported to anyone in authority in the organization where they occur (Rutter, 1996). The first step that must be taken when someone invades your space, touches you, or makes a suggestive remark, is to make a clear, direct verbal response: "I don't appreciate that." The harasser often feigns surprise and acts as though you are making something out of nothing. If you get such a reaction, stand your ground and describe very specifically what bothered you: "You were standing too close to me" or "I find your language offensive." It is important that you call attention to the inappropriate behavior early on, because studies show that harassment on the job is seldom a one-time occurrence. Sexual remarks and pressure for dates often go on for 6 months or more (Fitzgerald, 1993). If the harassing behavior continues, warn the individual that you may have to discuss the matter with his or her supervisor or with the human resources department. Many institutions now have someone designated to deal with cases of harassment. Keep written records of incidents and warnings that you have given. Include the names of witnesses to the egregious behavior. Send a registered letter to the offender asking that the harassment stop, keeping a file copy for yourself. If none of your initial limit-setting efforts are successful in stopping the harassment, filing a formal complaint or seeking legal counsel may be necessary. While going to court can be a time-consuming and expensive undertaking, many lawyers collect no fee if the case is lost or if there is no money awarded for damages. Do be aware of the Equal Employment Opportunity Commission's requirement that a complaint must be filed within either 180 or 300 days from the date of the incident, depending on the state where you live (Rutter, 1996). Of course, far better than these last-resort remedies would be prevention of the harassment in the first place. Its incidence will surely begin to decline when all nurses are the strong, empowered individuals that this book is devoted to developing.

IF YOU'RE THE RECIPIENT OF HORIZONTAL HOSTILITY

There are several ways to deal with the problem of horizontal hostility (discussed in Chapter 5), including direct confrontation of the other nurse as soon as you learn of his or her destructive gossip or sabotage. Luther Christman provides an example of another approach: using humor.

> *As many probably are aware, I was the first man in the profession to be appointed as a dean of nursing. Two years after this appointment I was attending a meeting of deans of nursing. After the opening plenary session, the dean of one of the major university schools walked to a floor microphone and asked everyone to remain until she made an important statement. She*

announced, "All those wonderful things you have heard about what is happening at Vanderbilt School of Nursing have nothing to do with Luther Christman's competence, because he doesn't have any. The only reason the programs are taking place is because every man on the entire faculty automatically gives in to any request he makes whenever he makes it." A dead and strained silence ensued as she stood at the microphone with her hands on her hips. I sensed the great uneasiness and moved to the floor microphone that was closest to me. Even though I was somewhat irked, I merely commented, "She just says that because it is true." Titters, then roars of laughter followed. The dean stood somewhat stunned and annoyed as everyone left the room. All those who approached me were jovial in their interactions with me.

Perceiving events with a humorous slant helps to keep blood pressure at normal levels. I had a very early experience that helped me understand behavior. When I was a first-year student in nursing, I established a pleasant relationship with the chief of psychiatry. One day I said to him, "Dr. Bond, you appear to be different from any other person in this hospital. I have never seen you upset or disturbed by anything that happens." He replied, "Young man, you too can be that way. Whenever I am interacting with other people, I always treat them as if they were paranoid schizophrenics. Who can become upset over what a paranoid schizophrenic says or does?" I have used this concept all my professional life and it has enabled me to be relaxed and not as irritated as many. A few months after that incident with the dean, I learned that that very morning she had been called into the chancellor's office and given five minutes to resign or be discharged. This helped explain why she had projected her anger at me.

IF YOUR TASK SEEMS IMPOSSIBLE

Distinguished nursing leader Angela Barron McBride has always seemed unflappable to me, calmly taking on the presidency of nursing's largest organization (Sigma Theta Tau) and, more recently, the deanship of the nation's largest nursing school (Indiana University). Through the years I have always looked forward to her addresses at professional meetings because she so freely shares the secrets of her success with others. But recently McBride faced what initially seemed to be an impossible task. She tells us of her anger and how she dispelled it:

I am a great believer in the extent to which explanations of events consequently shape feelings, behavior, and future expectations. When I became dean of Indiana University School of Nursing—one school of nursing but with offerings on eight campuses—I was angry not to find much of a paper trail in the files that described what was intended in the development of a so-called university school. I was expected to manage a structure that had only been vaguely defined, but required me to interact not only with a president, but [also] eight chancellors and eight academic vice-chancellors. I wanted principles spelled out to use in guiding future actions, and was angry that mine was an impossible task: to manage an entity about which there were no common agreements, either at the university or [at] school levels.

It is not uncommon for new administrators to want to bring down the furies of the gods on those who have gone before, and seem to have created what does not make sense by today's standards. The trouble with such anger is that it leaves one sulky instead of action-oriented. What helped me was to reconceptualize the situation.

First of all, what the university was experiencing was generally true for other schools operating university-wide. In a matrix organization where discipline interacts with campus mores, matters will never be clear because of the organizational complexity. Second, I began to see that the school was at a different developmental stage. The issue was no longer the establishment of basic programs but moving existing programs forward so they could address the needs of quickly changing health care delivery systems. I always feel better when I conceptualize a problem as generic or developmental rather than personal, because the former makes me feel as if I'm dealing with the issues of the day while the latter makes me feel negative about my institution and my own abilities. Finally, I came to realize that the university probably was only now ready to have the various chancellors, academic vice-chancellors, and nursing leaders go through the task of forging common understandings, because some trust had been established and we were now capable of higher-order thinking. Since one of my talents is bringing people together for a common purpose, I began to feel as if there might be a fit between my person and the place. My generalized anger began to dissipate as I got down to the task at hand.

IF YOU'RE WORKING WITH AN UNREASONABLE MANAGER

What if your problem is an unreasonable manager, supervisor, or dean? It is no secret that individuals with personality disorders and other kinds of mental pathology can and do achieve leadership positions in organizations. Having to work under such an individual can be pure hell. Here's one nurse's story:

Twice in my career I have been deeply involved in the removal of a key person in a school of nursing. In the first instance, the individual attempted the divide-and-conquer approach. She got the weakest members of the faculty on her side [by] showing favoritism. At the same time, she attempted to make life hell for those of us she perceived as threats or as strong persons. One favorite tactic was to call me into her office and scream at me. Needless to say, the stress was unbearable. Much as I was angry at the perpetrator of this misery, I was even angrier at colleagues who, behind her back, would go on and on about how bad things were but to her face, and to outside evaluators who were brought in, would say everything was wonderful. Six of us—three tenured and three nontenured—went to administration. I felt we stuck our necks out and then did not get support.

I decided, however, that it would be self-destructive to let the stress and anger eat at me, so I channeled it into scholarly work. I wrote a number of books [and] articles, did presentations, collaborated with clinical and academic colleagues on research projects. When it became clear that the top administration at the university was too afraid of the legislature to act, I made plans to leave. Having built up my scholarship, service, and teaching records significantly, I was able to use my work to negotiate for the position I wanted. Furthermore, among those of us who left, as well as those who stood strong, there grew a camaraderie and a feeling that justice would out eventually.

When a new president was appointed, he examined the data, looked at the accomplishments of those of us who had left, and acted swiftly to end the reign of terror. [I] not only [took] my integrity as a faculty member intact, but I also learned from the experience how to handle another, should it arise—and it did. The style was in some ways different, but many of the tactics were the same. This time I rallied all the tenured faculty and insisted that the only way we would eventually win would be to stand together. We did and the administration acted.

One of the most valuable tactics I learned was to turn negative energy and anger into positive activities. Second, I learned to consult wise persons from other disciplines. Third, I learned how to counter the divide-and-conquer tactics used by many destructive and insecure leaders. What was not so evident to me the first time around was crystal clear the second.

IF YOU LOSE YOUR JOB

What if the unthinkable happens and you find yourself the recipient of a pink slip? A few years ago during the nursing shortage, today's widespread layoffs and terminations could not have been imagined. Within my personal circle of acquaintances, the number of highly qualified nurses who have lost their jobs is shocking. One woman had been the CEO of a major mental health facility for 20 years but got the shaft during a merger. She wasn't even allowed to apply for her old job. For the first time in my lifetime, many nurses are job-scared. While I encourage each of you to do everything you can to make yourself indispensable to your organization and to obtain additional education, certifications, and other credentials to ensure your marketability if the unthinkable happens, no action on your part can be guaranteed to prevent losing your job.

Job terminations are occurring for a variety of reasons other than institutional reorganization and downsizing. Elizabeth Shogren was dismissed by her hospital after a back injury. The hospital administrators claimed that an RN should be able to lift 100 pounds, and, because she could not do this, they offered her a job as an admitting clerk. Shogren describes what it felt like to lose her job:

> *A whole lot of emotional turmoil goes on in addition to the physical pain of the injury. Nurses have integrated their role as an RN into their identity— nursing is an expression of who they are. This is more than a loss of a career. It's a loss of your core identity as a person. (Elizabeth Shogren, cited in Helmlinger, 1997, p. 66)*

Shogren spent 2 discouraging years looking for a nursing position before she went to work for the Minnesota Nurses Association. However, her story illustrates good problem-solving tactics. When other approaches were unsuccessful, she went to the courts. She sued the hospital on the basis of its offer of a job as admitting clerk, contending that this was not "suitable work" for a registered nurse. She won. The Minnesota Supreme Court ruled in her favor, resulting in an improved definition of "suitable work" for RNs that will benefit other nurses in the state.

Barry Adams was a whistleblower. He got his pink slip when he spoke out about his concerns about patient safety. He did all the right things when he went to meet with the director of nursing. He had the data to document errors and injury. But the director told him, "There are no unsafe work environments, only unsafe nursing practice" (Adams, 1997, p. 80). Adams was terminated for "insubordination." After he was fired, he filed a wrongful termination suit against the hospital. In a chilling coincidence, the same day that an article about Adams's lawsuit appeared in the *Boston Globe*, the newspaper also reported the accidental death of a patient at the hospital that had fired him. The nurse who had given the lethal morphine overdose had had no previous training in infusion pumps—exactly the dangerous kind of situation Adams had placed his job on the line to protest. Like Shogren, Adams is seeking resolution in the courts. His lawyer states, "If successful, Barry's case would be the first to clearly articulate the right of nurses to be protected from retribution for advocating on behalf of their patients" (Canavan, 1997c).

Ageism was the culprit in the next nurse's unfair termination. Internationally known nursing scholar and journal editor Phyllis Stern received a pink slip from her university at the age of 65. The Canadian Supreme Court had ruled that forced retirement is not a violation of an individual's rights, and the financially strapped university saw an opportunity to cut the faculty rolls with impunity. But Phyllis was not prepared for this development and not ready to retire. Having earned her doctorate in midlife, she was chronologically in midcareer and thriving on a busy schedule of teaching, research, and professional society leadership. Furthermore, she had not taught at the institution long enough to accrue a livable pension and feared running out of money in her forced retirement. To put it mildly, Phyllis was angry at becoming just a number—65. Here's what happened:

> *We got two weeks notice after the Supreme Court decision that our services would no longer be needed after June 30. Most faculty in Canadian universities are unionized, and mine was no exception. So I went to a union meeting, and here were nine old guys and the lone woman. Their chins were dragging on the table. They were feeling used up and cast out. I felt that way for about a week. But I found my mouth too crowded with my thumb stuck in it. So I got busy.*
>
> *Although I was a Canadian citizen, I had kept my U.S. citizenship. So unlike the nine old guys, I had options. I started calling around to my U.S. network. I looked at the ads, but glossed over most. I applied for a chair position at Indiana University–Purdue University, Indianapolis. I wasn't hot about living in Indianapolis, but my husband gave me his usual line, "Keep an open mind." Well, it turned out to be a nifty place, and I've been happier in this job than any I've had until now. I am the oldest person working here at the school. I'm still trying to decide what I want to be when I grow up.*

For each of these individuals, and for you, if you are a victim of downsizing or restructuring, the concept of transition is useful. The word means a change from one thing to another. Even when the change is viewed as positive (e.g., marriage, childbirth), there is a loss. We can never go back to the way things were. What do we know from research about transitions? Certainly, they are more difficult when they occur suddenly and you have no choice—like a pink slip with no warning. Transitions are also more difficult if you customarily view change as scary rather than challenging. And without a doubt, any transition will be more difficult if you do not have adequate support from significant others. The timing of events in relation to the life cycle is important too: A career transition will be more stressful if you are involved simultaneously in a midlife crisis (or in another of life's developmental transitions). Having undergone a number of life transitions, including the death of my parents, a midlife divorce, becoming a single parent, remarriage, and becoming a stepparent, as well as numerous career peregrinations, I have always taken comfort in John Sanford's (1977) maxim that all change requires the death of something in order that something new may develop.

One of the best empirical examinations of life transitions has been completed by Daniel Levinson (1978, 1996). Through in-depth study of the lives of men and women, he learned that the life structure evolves through a sequence of alternating stable periods and transitional periods. Each of the transitional periods ordinarily lasts about 5 years. Therefore, if you tally them up, almost half our adult lives is spent in transition (Levinson, 1996). If we can wrap our minds around this fact, I believe it is reassuring. Transitions are inevitable, and most of us endure them and grow because of them, even if initially the disruption was of great magnitude. After we complete the necessary tasks of terminating, questioning, and exploring new options, we build a new life structure that will serve us well—until the next transition.

As you problem-solve to deal with a job layoff or termination, this may be the time to consider a radically new career direction. If you have always been a provider of clinical services, perhaps you would enjoy teaching. A huge nursing faculty shortage is predicted in just a few years. Or perhaps the prospects of doing research sound appealing. It's not too late for you to go to graduate school. I teach students who are in their 30s, 40s, and 50s every day. They are excited about their new trajectory. The demand for master's and doctoral nurses will be twice the supply available in 2000 (U.S. Department of Health and Human Services, 1990b). You might also consider opening an independent practice. More and more nurses are doing so.

IF OTHERS ARE NOT RESPONSIVE TO CONCERNS ABOUT A PATIENT

Advocating on behalf of a patient is an important aspect of good nursing. In earlier chapters, we included some short vignettes in which anger empowered nurses to go to bat for their patients. The following is a longer, more complex account, involving anger not only at the patient's doctors but also at his nurses, and requiring a number of strategies on the part of this nurse. First, she explains the problem:

The patient was in cardiac intensive care with complications after open heart surgery. A protracted hospitalization involving postoperative bleeding, a nosocomial infection, and extended ventilator dependence left him anxious and depressed. Part of my anger was related to staff who seemed to have a much lower idea of a standard of care than I did. For instance, immediately after surgery, the clinical specialist called the family to say "he is okay," and was ready to hang up. When I said we needed more details about blood loss and the surgical procedures, the clinical specialist had no idea and did not propose to do anything else. My anger grew as staff skipped some informed consents, ignored suggestions for a communication board for the vent-dependent patient, disregarded the need to treat anxiety and depression, and failed to order some important lab tests. When I asked the staff what communication aids they used for these patients, they thought a communication board was a good idea. They said they used to have one, but it disappeared. I was irritated when staff did not explain problems to the patient. The patient became more depressed as the surgical team delayed removing the ET tube, never clarifying why, and avoided speaking with him for several days.

The nurse used diverse tactics to problem-solve on this patient's behalf:

I've rarely been so angry that colleagues did not provide a standard of care, and yet I needed to contain the anger and negotiate with staff to improve patient care. In several instances [when] the proposed action seemed unwise, I asked the professionals for their rationale so I could explain it to the patient. This was effective because often I was told, "This is what we do," and I could inquire about their procedures for individualizing care. Initially I offered suggestions, such as the communication board. Although staff thought this a good idea, nothing happened. I then brought the patient paper and pen. Next I wanted to address the patient's anxiety. I gathered necessary data and determined the best person to approach. The chief resident did agree to order medications, but ordered oral medications and did not order the necessary Haldol until the patient's agitation and confusion prompted him to pull out the tubes.

I ignored the small frustrations and focused on the patient's major issues, and I worked to form alliances with the staff. All the consultants encouraged removal of the ET tube, but they seemed impotent. I confronted the surgical team because the patient wanted the tube removed, but the surgeons avoided him and failed to do so. After paging, leaving messages, and other attempts to speak with the surgeon, I decided to stay with the patient until rounds. However, the evening RN asked me to leave. I agreed, provided that she would communicate the patient's wishes to the surgeon. She replied that she did not think she could. I stared at her in amazed silence and anger. I did not raise my voice as I said, "You do not believe it is the nurse's role to advocate and communicate for a patient on a ventilator?

I conveyed the patient's distress and frustration to the surgical resident, and asked that the surgeons talk with him daily and provide a clear answer about when the ET tube would be removed. After this, the surgical team did talk with him daily, but days passed without explaining to the patient the continued ET tube. The surgeon refused my request for a team conference with family, surgeons, and consultants. The patient lost about 1/5 of his body weight before finally, after much nudging, nutritional supplements were ordered. And finally, the surgeons agreed to extubate, oxygenation was adequate, a defective ET tube was discovered, and the patient left intensive care.

Although this nurse, through constant vigilance and persistent advocacy, was able to get staff to address her concerns, what other avenues are available to you? If you fail to resolve a concern about patient care quality or safety through workplace channels, what can you do? Your options include filing a complaint with your state's board of nursing, department of health, insurance commissioner, or elected representatives (look in the state government pages of your telephone book). Written complaints can also be made to the Joint Commission for Accreditation of Health Care Organizations. The address is 1 Renaissance Blvd., Oakbrook Terrace, Illinois, 60181. Be sure to document inadequate staffing, unsafe practices, accidents, injuries, and missed treatments; make notes about dates, times, and personnel. You can report potential problems as well as actual ones. Send a copy of your written complaint to your state nurses association to assist them in tracking problems (American Nurses Association, 1995).

IF ACTION BY AN INDIVIDUAL IS NOT ENOUGH

Some problems cannot be solved by individual action; the power of the collective is required to make a strong impact. In such situations, nurses must unite in coalitions to lobby, persuade, and negotiate. The power of nurse unity was clearly demonstrated in recent events at Boston's Brigham and Women's Hospital. The hospital's 1,900 nurses are organized in a bargaining unit of the Massachusetts Nurses Association, and their unit has a track record of successfully negotiating for them. But in August 1996, the contract negotiations, after nearly a year, were hopelessly bogged down and a strike seemed inevitable. Nurses' morale had plummeted as workplace conditions significantly deteriorated, but no one knew if these nurses could unite to take the radical step of walking out on strike on October 1. They had never gone on strike before. Some felt that striking was unprofessional. Emergency department nurse Karen Daley (1997) tells what happened:

> *Mandatory overtime, inadequate staffing, elimination of permanent RN positions lost through attrition, increased use of per diems throughout the hospital, and the practice of floating RNs to other areas with no formal orientation were all too commonplace. These conditions jeopardized our ability to provide safe, effective nursing care. . . . The solidarity we felt . . . as the strike vote approached was equivalent . . . to drawing a line in the sand for hospital administration. That line was drawn solidly as 1,200 [85% of voting bargaining unit members] voted to strike. The next day, hundreds of nurses turned out in a downpour to carry signs for several hours in an informational picket. Two days later, a marathon 19-hour negotiating session resulted in a tentative contract agreement that included most of the bargaining unit proposals and language and was later overwhelmingly ratified by the membership. (p. 80)*

I applaud the unity and courage of the nurses at Brigham and Women's Hospital. Whether or not you support collective bargaining, and I know some nurses view it as "unprofessional," you must admit that it gave the nurses in this situation clout that they would not otherwise have had. I am a firm believer in joining together in professional organizations to build a base of power. I will be very specific here and state my own conviction that every single nurse should join the American Nurses Association. The fragmentation of nurse power into a multiplicity of organizations keeps us from speaking with one strong voice. If you don't like the positions that the ANA is taking, let your voice be heard within its deliberations, not outside it. If you don't want to come to meetings, send your dues money to contribute to the work that the association does on your behalf. Roberts (1983) attributed nurses' lack of participation in their professional organizations to the self-hatred that is common in oppressed groups. Because nurses do not feel proud or powerful, they refuse to join with others whom they perceive as powerless. They have internalized their oppressors' view of them.

Fortunately, efforts are going forward on a number of fronts as this book is going to press. To combat the dangerous delegation of professional nursing activities to UAPs (unlicensed assistive personnel), the ANA and the state associations have taken the message "When you cut nurses, the patient bleeds" to Congress, the media, and consumer groups. The ANA is also lobbying to discourage state boards from changing their practice acts. There was a close call in Montana, but the Montana Nurses Association prevailed. The state board of nursing there had tried to lift restrictions on the types of tasks that could be delegated to UAPs. The proposed rules would have allowed nurses to delegate anything that could be "safely" done by an aide. The scary aspect is that if nurses give away their tasks, the patient loses the benefit of the complex nursing assessment and decision-making process that should accompany the tasks. In fact, we should stop using the word *tasks*, because it's too easy for hospital administrators to think in simplistic terms of substituting one worker for another to perform them. In locales where this simplistic reasoning has been used to permit UAPs to perform work that RNs should be doing, patient deaths are already taking place (see Chapter 1).

Getting back to the Montana story, the state nurses association vigorously opposed lifting restrictions on delegation to UAPs and had numerous meetings with the board of nursing to explain its concerns. At last, the board dropped its ill-conceived idea, leaving the current rules unchanged. Barbara Booher, the Montana Nurses Association's executive director, had this to say about the successful lobbying effort: *"I know nurses are known for trying to be accommodating and making a variety of situations work where no other profession gives their practice away to this extent. And I was glad that in Montana we were able to get that message across"* (Booher, cited in Canavan, 1997b, p. 58).

To buttress nursing's contention that patient outcomes are directly related to the number of RNs on staff, the ANA commissioned a study. Data were collected from 502 hospitals. Study findings provide hard evidence that higher RN staffing is correlated with shorter length of stay for patients and lower incidence of preventable conditions such as postoperative infections, pneumonia, and pressure ulcers (Canavan, 1997d). Additional data are being collected in a number of states (California, Arizona, Minnesota, North Dakota, Texas, and Virginia) to substantiate that higher RN staffing results in lower rates of adverse patient outcomes. This empirical evidence will be invaluable in our ongoing efforts to demonstrate the value of professional nursing care. Work has also begun by the President's Advisory Commission on Consumer Protection and Quality in the Health Care Industry, which will draft a Consumer Bill of Rights. Three nurses, including the ANA president, are involved in the work of this commission. And there is legislation in the works to protect whistleblowers like Barry Adams who speak out about unsafe conditions for patients. The 42,000 nurse members who have volunteered to serve on the ANA's N-STAT (Nurses Strategic Action Team) are working hard to mobilize grassroots support for the Patient Safety Act, which will safeguard nurses from employer retribution for whistleblowing.

THE BUTTERFLY EFFECT

In a rut of apathy and cynicism, some nurses feel that the actions of one individual cannot possibly make a difference. Let me remind you of the butterfly effect. When a butterfly moves its wings deep in the Amazon forest, tiny air currents result. These currents affect larger eddies, and circumstance compounds circumstance, until the barely perceptible movement of that particular butterfly at that particular time changes the course—weeks later—of a tornado (Leach, 1990). I think of human examples like Rosa Parks, who refused to move to the back of the bus where African-Americans were assigned to sit: one woman, one act of quiet protest against the idiocy of racist seat assignment in a public bus. I also think of Rosli Naf, whose name is not nearly so well known as that of Rosa Parks. Naf was a Swiss Red Cross nurse. She was 30 years old when she was sent to Nazi-occupied France in 1941 to care for 100 Jewish children and adults. Naf had never had contact with Jews and had heard much anti-Semitic propaganda about them in Switzerland, but she quickly came to love the children and was horrified when 42 of the teenagers were forcibly taken away to a transit camp that was a stop on the way to the Auschwitz death camp. Over the next 2 days, she made her way by bicycle, bus, and taxi to the transit camp. She marched in and began to badger the guards to release the children. She got them out of the camp but was refused permission to take them to safety in

Switzerland. So Naf decided that she must help the youngsters escape. She made them fake IDs and gave them train fare, having arranged an escape route with the help of the French underground and some Swiss citizens. The first five teenagers were caught at the French-Swiss border. Two served jail time but survived, but the other three were sent to Auschwitz, where they were gassed. The rest made it to safety. Naf was fired for her actions because she acted without Red Cross approval. Years later, when interviewed in a Swiss nursing home, her only regret was that she was not able to save more children: one woman, one courageous act during the insanity of the Holocaust (Kelley, 1997).

All of us who learn of Rosa Parks and Rosli Naf are profoundly affected and inspired by their heroism. Likewise, the assertive actions of one nurse in his or her workplace can become linked to the empowering actions of other nurses. We, and the butterfly, are part of the organic whole of the universe. Not all of us will display the uncommon heroism of Rosa Parks and Rosli Naf, nor will all of us run for political office or work at the national level in our professional organizations. But what we do each day, blooming where we are planted, *can* make a difference. The psychologist and philosopher William James once said:

> *I am done with great things and big things, with great institutions and big success. And I am for those tiny, invisible molecular forces that work from individual to individual, creeping through the crannies of the world like so many soft rootlets, or like the capillary oozing of water; but which, given time, will rend the hardest monuments of men's pride.*

12

Dreaming the Future of Nursing

> Heal the past, live the present,
> dream the future.
>
> Mary Walker, PhD, RN, FAAN, from a speech given
> October 11, 1996 at the University of Tennessee

What is your dream of nursing's future? As the 21st century approaches, futuristic prognostications about health care fill the pages of both professional and popular books and magazines. Let's look at a few of the more intriguing predictions that are being made. Uwe Rheinhart, a Princeton health economist, says that the age of specialization is over. He predicts that the LPN is going to be doing the work of the RN, the RN is going to be doing the work of the physician, the GP is going to be doing the work of the specialist, and the specialist is going to be driving taxicabs (Rheinhart, cited in Cummings, 1996).

Columbia University's Eli Ginzberg asserts that managed care cannot sustain its current growth and industry dominance. Furthermore, it will be unable to answer the needs of the American people for universal coverage, sustainable financing, and better care (Ginzberg, 1997; Ginzberg & Ostow, 1997). As the profit-oriented practices of managed care plans—such as delaying authorization of life-saving treatments because of cost—have been exposed, public concern has grown. Articles like *Time's* "Backlash Against HMOs" (Church, 1997) are appearing in the popular press. Ginzberg also highlights the fallacy that managed care is cutting costs: During the years of managed care's rapid ascendance, health care costs have not decreased but rather quadrupled (from $250 billion in 1980 to $1 trillion in 1995).

A variety of nursing leaders offered their visions in a recent *Image* article entitled "Future of Nursing Scholarship" (1997). Here's a sampling. Jean Watson, who directs the Center for Human Caring at the University of Colorado, believes that the next era promises the emergence of a "mature Nightingale model of nursing," which allows nursing to return to its spiritual roots. Sheila Ryan, the dean of nursing at University of Rochester, predicts that we will move from hierarchical bureaucracies, organizations, and professions to horizontal-matrix organizations and teams of disciplines. Norma Lang, the dean of nursing at the University of Pennsylvania, foresees the increased use of telemedicine, telehealth, and telenursing for teaching nursing students and patients, as well as for diagnosis and follow-up.

Jennifer Jenkins, a nurse who is the vice president of Healthcare Concepts in Memphis, envisions new nursing positions in the next century: manager of networks of patients through information systems, holistic healer, geriatric ombudsman, nurse architect, nurse engineer, cyber educator, nurse energist, personal healing guide, and mall manager (Jenkins, 1996). Most of these are self-explanatory, but you may not realize that by mall manager Jenkins means a nurse-managed Internet mall that provides health-oriented products and services. As she explains it, this "one-stop-shop permits a new mother to receive coaching on breast feeding, a drug addict to find an acupuncture detox treatment program and a ninety-year-old couple [to] find a nurse-supervised trip into the backcountry of Yellowstone National Park to do some fly fishing" (Jenkins, 1996, p. 19).

Relative to most other health professions, the value of nurses will rise over the next 10 years, according to Peter Buerhaus (Buerhaus, cited in *Nursing Leadership in the 21st Century*, 1996). He predicts that "this will occur even if nothing remarkable is done to change clinical practice, education, or leadership capacities. However, if the profession changes in ways that enable nurses to better respond to the needs of purchasers, employers, and society, there is much potential for the value of nurses to rise at a rate unprecedented in the history of the profession. . . . There will be more opportunities available for nurses than they can take advantage."

May Wykle envisions the nurse of the future as the "hub in the wheel" as manager and coordinator of all providers instrumental in promoting the health of the population (Wykle, cited in *Nursing Leadership in the 21st Century*, 1996).

Here are my predictions. We are certainly in for a dizzying roller-coaster ride of changes, some of them unwanted and unpleasant. But we're going to ride it out and avail ourselves of the new opportunities described by Jenkins, Buerhaus, and others. The public will demand that the federal government break up corporate monopolies in health care. There will no longer be insurance companies that also own health maintenance organizations, hospitals, and drug manufacturers. Currently there are 56 laws pending in 35 states and more than a dozen pieces of pending federal legislation that pertain to regulation of the health care system. Wasteful administrative costs—such as the enormous salaries, bonuses, and stock options paid to executives of HMOs and for-profit hospitals—will be curtailed drastically. Reengineering will be regarded as a costly flop. Already, the reengineering gurus who launched the personnel cutbacks of the mid-1990s are backpedaling. Michael Hammer, one of the leaders of the movement, has acknowledged that he and other movement leaders "forgot about people" (cited in L. Thomas, 1996). In a remarkable admission of naivete, Hammer admitted that he had been "insufficiently appreciative of the human dimension." The newspaper article quoted him as saying, "I've learned that's critical." What he didn't understand is the anger, demoralization, and burnout that survivors feel when their colleagues are canned. The survivors of the cutbacks resist management's pressure to increase productivity—the "speedups" we talked about in Chapter 1. Ultimately, then, downsizing does not result in saving the organization money. Productivity cannot be emphasized to the exclusion of consideration for workers. There's another new term—for those companies whose bones were picked clean by the reengineering experts—"corporate anorexia." Many health care organizations that greedily gobbled up the concept of "lean and mean" are hiring again. And guess what? Some observers of the national scene are actually predicting a nursing shortage in the future. In a January 20, 1997 article, *Time* magazine listed nursing as one of the 15 hottest fields, with a projected growth of 473,000 jobs by 2005.

A heyday for nurse entrepreneurs is coming. More and more nurses will be presidents of their own businesses—everything from hospices, adult day care establishments, fitness emporiums, and holistic healing retreat centers, to software design firms and consulting firms of all types. Community nursing organizations (CNO's) will contract to provide primary care for groups of patients. Such organizations are already proving their worth in four Medicare demonstration projects funded by the Health Care Financing Administration. In a CNO, members are assigned to a nurse who works with them on health promotion or manages existing problems. The nurse may meet with them in a clinic, community center, or their homes. Data on costs and quality of care are currently being analyzed, but preliminary results show reduced hospitalization and emergency department visits as well as high member satisfaction (Schraeder, Lamb, Shelton, & Britt, 1997). These results should not surprise us, for after all, nurses know more about holistic health and wellness than any other group of professionals and excel at management of chronic diseases and elder care.

Let's not forget the acutely ill. Hospitals will always need highly skilled nurses because they are going to become giant intensive care units. Unlicensed assistive personnel cannot be safely utilized for direct patient care in such facilities. One hospital has already been fined $25,000 by the Indiana State Department of Health for failing to have enough nurses on duty (Cahill, 1997). In the year 2005, a large percentage of RNs (57.4%) will still be employed in hospitals (Shindul-Rothschild et al., 1996). But these nurses will also do home visits to the patients they cared for in the hospital, and other changes in acute care nursing practice are likely.

There will be greater gender balance in the profession. Educators are seeing a sharp increase in interest among men; enrollment figures have doubled (Fagin, 1994). When I look out at a roomful of students to deliver a lecture, men are sprinkled throughout the lecture hall. It's nice to see. Many midlife men are choosing nursing as a second career, and not all young men are finding the get-your-MBA-and-then-a-BMW route appealing. As the numbers of men and women equalize, men will not feel marginalized, excluded from the female "sorority," as one of our research participants phrased it. There is some evidence that the social isolation of men in nursing is already decreasing, as shown in new research by one of our doctoral graduates, Stephen Krau. He compared loneliness of female nurses, male nurses, and male ministers (ministers served as a comparison group of men in a helping profession that is traditionally male). No statistically significant differences were found between groups, refuting previous indications that loneliness is a problem for men who choose nursing as a career.

Nurses will exhibit a new pride in who they are and what they do. Whether they are CEOs, family nurse practitioners (FNPs), or staff nurses, they will feel confident in their knowledge and comfortable in marketing their expertise. Workplaces will not be free of stress, but nurses will be hardier and more stress-resistant. The American Nurses Association will be more than a million strong, and will be one of the most powerful political action committees in the nation's capital. Nurse researchers will be cited in the daily newspapers as frequently as medical researchers.

Nurses will form new partnerships with psychologists, social workers, and other professionals. Having my PhD in psychology, I have a long-standing interest in collaboration between nurses and psychologists and have written on the topic (Thomas, 1996). An example of such collaboration appeared in a recent Internet message from a Wyoming psychologist named Michael Enright (federal-ppa@lists.apa.org, March 15, 1997) who is studying to become a nurse practitioner. He was only marginally involved, as a consultant, in this story, but relates it with pride because of the excellent care provided by the patient's psychologist and her nurse practitioner. The patient was a 13-year-old girl hospitalized by the psychologist after a suicide attempt (psychologists have had admitting privileges at the hospital for 15 years). The patient's care was jointly managed by the psychologist and the nurse practitioner. Her symptoms prior to admission had included labile moods, lethargy (with intermittent episodes of agitation, in which she cut her forearms with a razor blade), and hair loss. Lab tests for thyroid dysfunction such as T3, T4, and TSH were normal. It was only when the nurse practitioner suspected a rare form of hypothyroidism (Wilson's disease) and ordered additional tests, that the patient was correctly diagnosed. She responded dramatically to thyroid supplementation and went from suicide precautions to discharge overnight. The nurse's diagnostic skills and intervention were superb. The psychologist played a pivotal role in working with the patient and her family during the dramatic emotional and psychological changes.

My final prediction? All nurses will share their expertise and concern in the communities where they live. They will be heavily involved in health councils, citizens groups, and politics. They will wield their power in the board room and at the ballot box. Virginia Henderson once said, "It seems hardly possible to me that an excellent nurse can be at the same time an indifferent or socially inexperienced citizen."

EXTINCTION? NOT A CHANCE!

Some years ago I wrote a futuristic story about Joey, a child hospitalized in the year 2040 after the profession of nursing had become extinct (Thomas, 1980). Joey was cared for in an efficient, fully computerized facility with a fleet of efficient, speedy technicians. But he was lonely and quite delighted when Grandma, a former nurse, came to visit. Enthralled, he listened as she told him about nurses (he had never heard of them). "What happened to nurses, Grandma? Why don't we have them anymore?" asked Joey. Grandma looked sad, and maybe a little bitter too. She was slow in formulating her answer, as if, after all this time, she still could not understand what had happened: "I guess nurses couldn't decide what they were and what they wanted to do, Joey. They just couldn't get together . . . organizations held conferences, conventions, meetings, seminars, task forces, and workshops. But after all the talking, there was still no agreement on anything. . . . No one listened to anyone else, Joey. People were too emotionally upset. . . . And while all of this was going on, technicians took care of the patients. Eventually, nurses weren't needed anymore. The end was really not very dramatic; as a matter of fact, everyone just forgot about nurses. To use the words of a 20th century poet named Eliot, nursing ended 'not with a bang but a whimper.' "

I wrote the story, of course, as a wake-up call to you, my colleagues, not a prediction of what would actually come to pass. Neither then, nor now, have I been pessimistic about nursing's prospects for the future. Nurses are not an endangered species *if we unite*. History shows that when groups are threatened by outside forces, they become more cohesive within their own ranks. I have the privilege of teaching the individuals who will be the profession's leaders in the next century, and I can tell you that they are a fantastic cohort of men and women. They are critical thinkers and competent, creative caregivers. They are excited and proud to contemplate taking part in nursing's bright new future. They fill me with hope. But *all of us* are in charge of our future. Like Nightingale, we must tackle obstacles with determination, adopting her conviction that "never to know that you are beaten is the way to victory" (Nightingale, cited in Cook, 1913).

Conclusion

> The seeds of wisdom, peace, and wholeness
> are within each of our difficulties.
>
> Jack Kornfield 1993, p. 80

Although this book plumbed nurses' collective difficulties and private suffering, I do believe that wisdom, peace, and wholeness are possible. Nurses will get through this chaotic period. The practice of nursing will always be needed by society and will always attract individuals who have a vocation to give loving care. In fact, the latest national survey of 2 million high school juniors showed that nursing ranked third out of the 65 most preferred career choices (*Occupational Outlook Quarterly,* cited in *Newsline,* 1997). Nursing yields great joys. That is why so many of us remain devoted to it, even though we've been "ordered to care in a society that [does] not value caring," as historian Susan Reverby (1987) has argued. I asked some nurses to share what keeps them enthused about this profession, and this is what they said:

When asked why I've stayed in nursing for the past 27 years I can look at this past week as an example of what keeps me going. I cared for a 49-year-old mother dying of lung cancer and a 35-year-old mother with advanced breast cancer, playing a role in helping both of these women come to terms with their disease. Two weeks ago we thought both of them would not survive more than a week or two. Both women were frightened and unable to talk about what was happening with their families. The other oncology nurses and I worked with these patients and their families to help them share their feelings and to understand what was happening to them. The patient with lung cancer died days ago surrounded by family and friends. The breast cancer patient received a new chemotherapeutic agent and responded! Her liver function improved dramatically, she became more alert, and is going home today. No one knows how much time this response will give her, but she'll be at home with her husband and children for a little while. Two years ago this drug was not available and she would surely have died. Oncology nursing has blessed me with the opportunity to have so many special caring relationships over the years. I've learned to accept death and help those facing it and at the same time to continually see the fantastic progress in the prevention, detection and treatment of cancer giving so many the gift of life. I can't think of any other profession that offers the intellectual stimulation and challenge along with the opportunity to relate to so many people in so many situations. I'm challenged and rewarded intellectually and emotionally every day. (Peggy Pierce)

I think of that woman who was so grateful that she could get a reliable method of birth control or the scared pregnant adolescent who didn't know what to do next. I remember the teenage couple who [were] so afraid that their new baby's cord had become infected. And the 150 older members of the community who brought their smiles and stories of earlier times with them to get their flu shots. And all those parents who brought their children for gamma globulin after they had been exposed to hepatitis at their day care. These are the things that make my anger fade. I forget about my feelings of powerlessness. I know that I make a difference. (Belinda McCall)

I am a person who needs to know that what I do makes a difference. Nursing has met this need for almost 40 years. I remember the wrenching pain of being with an elderly man on discharge day [when] we both knew he was going home to die. I remember the student who sat at my office door early one morning waiting to tell me she was pregnant. I have always been inspired by other nurses. Nurses are not compensated commensurate with the contribution they make to the nation's health. Luckily for society, nurses are motivated more by satisfaction than by the bottom line. Nursing makes me proud. It is a rare privilege for me to know I am part of a worldwide force that exists to improve the quality of people's lives. Nursing is who I am. (Carol Seavor)

I was only 5 years old when I decided I wanted to be a nurse. I did not have support from my family; quite the contrary. They told me that I did not have the physical, intellectual, or character strength to meet this goal. They thought that nursing embodied a life of drudgery, and furthermore, they were convinced I would not succeed. . . . I received a 3-year scholarship to a diploma program when I was 17. . . . At only one point in my life did I think of changing careers; this was when I received my first master's degree in child development. I continued my life in nursing because of the variety of experience that nursing offered and because of the soul satisfaction it brought to me. Through the years I have never lost my enthusiasm for assisting families to whatever level of wellness they are capable of. . . . Given the present climate in which females are socialized to believe that all professional avenues are open to them, I ask myself the obvious question: would I still choose nursing? My answer is a resounding "yes." (Patricia Droppleman)

Compare the testimony of these nurses about "making a difference" and "soul satisfaction" with the rueful remark of Michele Proto, a subject in the study by Levinson (1996) who has spent her career in business:

I wish I had a feeling that what I do is important. My work is geared toward making a lot of rich people richer. There is not one social benefit in anything I do, not one redeeming thing. Let's face it, there are no redeeming factors. What the hell am I doing this for? My tombstone will read: "She delivered projects on schedule." (p. 399)

Nursing, with all its stress and frustrations, is still a wonderful way to make a living. I have never once regretted choosing nursing in 1957. My nursing work has been a hugely important part of my life, bringing me great pleasure and satisfaction. Although I have done a number of different things—including med-surg floor nursing, inpatient and outpatient psychiatric nursing, administration, research, journal editing, and teaching students at the diploma, baccalaureate, master's, and doctoral levels—I've enjoyed each and every one of them. What a marvelous profession that so many different directions can be taken as one's interests change through the years! I've worked different shifts. I've been employed in places where I had to clock in and in places where I had academic freedom. I've worked in uniform and in street clothes, with lab coat and without. I've been poorly paid and well paid. I've toiled alongside humble nurse's aides who exemplified dignity and compassion as well as stellar leaders of the profession who shared their sophisticated theories, vision, and political savvy. I've nursed innocents and murderers. I've sat on dilapidated sofas in drug-infested housing projects and plush chairs in tastefully decorated board rooms. I've made mistakes as well as contributions. But I've *never* been bored or burned out. I plan to remain active in nursing until at least 2010—and beyond, if I still have my wits about me (I've asked several trusted friends to notify me if I begin to "lose it" and don't have enough sense to realize it). I hope to be there as we step into the new millennium because I want to see nursing's dreams of the future become actuality.

Just as I began this book, drawing inspiration from Nightingale's admonition to "Charge on," so also let me close with her inspiring words about doing all that we do as professional nurses as well as it can be done. Nightingale was quite demanding of herself as well as others. She yearned for others to share her passion, urgency, and commitment to better health for all people. Her standards for nursing were exacting. Out of 1,000 to 2,000 applicants to the Nightingale Training School each year, she selected only 15 to 30 students of the highest moral character (Smith, 1981). She viewed the graduates of the school as "nursing missioners" and kept up a voluminous correspondence with them as they sailed off to America, France, Australia, and the far corners of the earth to start new schools and upgrade nursing. In her missives to them, she continually exhorted them to display the highest professionalism and devotion to the art of nursing. Even though there was a nursing shortage in her time, Nightingale adamantly insisted that individuals with inferior preparation could not be substituted for educated nurses—even those with good intentions. "There is no such thing as amateur nursing," said Nightingale (Monteiro, 1985, p. 184). We still carry her legacy into the minds and hearts of people everywhere when we deliver superb professional nursing care. We must continue to fight for the rights of all people to have access to that care. Let us dedicate our efforts to our founder, who said:

The professional motive is the desire and perpetual effort to do the thing as well as it can be done, which exists just as much in the Nurse, as in the Astronomer in search of a new star, or in the Artist completing a picture. (Nightingale, cited in Nash, 1931, p. 271)

Epilogue

I realize that some of my readers would like to have more detail about the anger research alluded to in this book. In 1989 I put together a 14-member research team (all female, all nurses except for one psychologist) to conduct a descriptive study of women's anger. Unlike previous studies of women aroused to anger in artificial laboratory experiments or deeply troubled women discovering long-buried anger in psychotherapy, our study aimed to examine anger in everyday situations at home and at work. We wanted to know what provoked women's anger and how they expressed or inhibited it. Given the scant research and conflicting advice about anger management in both professional and popular literature, we wanted to know what ways of dealing with anger were health-promoting. There was plenty of advice about health-damaging thoughts and behaviors, but virtually no data-based information about constructive anger.

Data were collected over a 3-year period in a variety of community settings, including work sites, schools, and women's organizations. More than 500 women, between the ages of 25 and 66, participated in this initial phase of the study. The women represented a wide range of educational backgrounds, marital status, occupations, and income brackets. The racial composition of the sample closely approximated the racial composition of the U.S. population, with the exception of fewer Hispanics. Seventy-five of the women were nurses, and we found that the nurses, along with other human service professionals, scored highest among occupational groups on overall anger proneness.

Phase I of the Women's Anger Study was primarily quantitative. We used well-established and validated questionnaires to measure the anger variables, as well as other variables related to anger, such as stress, self-esteem, and depression. The test battery included Spielberger's Trait

Anger Scale, the Framingham Anger Scales, the Cognitive-Somatic Anger Scale, the Perceived Stress Scale, Rosenberg's Self-Esteem Scale, the Beck Depression Inventory, the Current Health Scale from Ware's Health Perceptions Questionnaire, Norbeck's Social Support Questionnaire, and a researcher-developed questionnaire assessing health indicators and demographics. There was a small qualitative component of the study, consisting of open-ended questions about the precipitants of women's anger, its targets, and its duration. Study participants wrote their responses to these questions. The Phase I findings were reported in the book *Women and Anger,* published in 1993 by Springer Publishing.

The second phase of the Women's Anger Study took place over the next 4 years and involved collection of several data sets from specific groups of women. What prompted further study was the need to know more about the context in which anger episodes occurred and the meaning of these experiences for women. The large quantitative investigation had provided useful data—quite useful, in fact, because our study was the first large, comprehensive examination of women's anger. But we found the written responses to our questions about anger incidents tantalizing in their brevity. We needed to conduct in-depth interviews with women to obtain richer, more complete descriptions of the anger incidents. Therefore, we chose phenomenology as our method.

Because Phase II was a phenomenological study, it differed significantly from Phase I with regard not only to method but also to sample size and other aspects. Details of the method may be found in our published papers. Interviews were conducted by members of the research team with 29 Caucasian women, ranging in age from 20s to 60s. Illustrative occupations ranged from homemaker, student, and waitress to business executive, college professor, and human service professional. Participants were selected on the basis of having experienced the phenomenon of anger and being willing to discuss it at length. Findings of this study are forthcoming in an article in *Journal of Advanced Nursing* (Thomas et al., in press). Because we had collected data only from Caucasian women, we embarked almost immediately on recruitment of a sample of African-American women. In-depth phenomenological interviews were subsequently conducted by two African-American members of our research team with nine women. Preliminary findings from this study were reported in 1997 at meetings of the Southern Nursing Research Society and the American Psychological Association, and the paper is in press at *Issues in Mental Health Nursing.*

In both of these samples of women, there were some nurses. Again, as we had seen with the quantitative data, it was clear that nurses were very angry. Although data from the nurse interviews were not pulled out for separate analysis, I was struck and disturbed by nurses' distress and powerlessness. I felt the need to focus more specifically on individuals in my own profession. Because the earlier studies were not designed solely to investigate work-related anger, a new data collection seemed advisable. Therefore, the Nurses Anger Study was launched and new interviews conducted. In conjunction with my colleague Pat Droppleman and doctoral student Marilyn Smith, data from nine female registered nurses were collected and analyzed. The sample included staff nurses, nurse managers, nurse practitioners, a midwife, and a nursing instructor. Educational preparation of the nurses ranged from AD to PhD, ages from 29 to 56, and years of practice from 7 to 34 years. Two participants were African-American and seven were Caucasian. Findings of this study were reported in *Nursing Forum* (Smith et al., 1996).

We still did not feel that we had finished examining nurses' anger, because we had not studied any men. At that time we were fortunate to have a male master's student, Aaron Brooks, who wanted to work with us to fulfill his research requirement. He was excited about interviewing men about their anger. Almost immediately, we launched the next project, which involved five male nurse participants. Their ages ranged from 28 to 38 and their nursing experience from 3 to 17 years. One nurse had a master's degree, two a bachelor's, one a diploma, and one an associate's degree. Findings of this study were also reported in *Nursing Forum* (Brooks et al., 1996).

Altogether, we have accumulated a vast amount of data on nurses. We have approximately five hundred pages of interview transcripts from registered nurses whose present or past work settings include intensive care, coronary care, behavioral health, orthopedics, neurology, oncology, med-surg, home health, primary care, long-term care, maternity, and public health. These nurses have held a variety of staff, management, and teaching positions, and some were in advanced practice roles such as nurse practitioner and clinical specialist. While we would not claim that we had a sample representative of the population of American nurses, it was certainly a diverse sample. You, the readers, can judge the validity of our findings. In phenomenology, a study is considered valid if it provides a compelling, thorough description of the phenomenon. Validity is further substantiated if the findings resonate with readers' own experience of anger in the workplace. There is a criterion called "fittingness" that is met when the findings of a study "fit" contexts other than the study situation and when people in those contexts view them as applicable to their experience (Sandelowski, 1986).

Members of the research team certainly found that nurses' stories were similar to our own lived experience. Analyzing the data aroused strong emotion. For nearly a year, members of the research team grappled with the pain of our study participants as the transcripts were read aloud and discussed. The nurses' words hung in the air, and our stomachs knotted as we listened to them. We resonated with the pain because we too had been in the hostile environment they described. We too had sometimes screamed, or seethed silently because we dared not speak. It was hard to set aside our own biases, as the method of phenomenology requires. For that reason, we took many of the interviews to an interdisciplinary phenomenology research group for assistance with the data analysis. We also took the final thematic structure back to some of our participants to ascertain if we had accurately captured their experience. Many encouraged us to publish something that would help nurses when we finished the research.

I became convinced that beyond reporting our research findings there was a moral imperative to propose strategies for channeling nurses' anger into positive interventions. That is, of course, the purpose of this book. I am also doing many talks and workshops for groups of nurses. Research is ongoing. As always, there are new questions and new directions to take. We plan to conduct a separate analysis of the data from the African-American nurses. Although we have used excerpts from their transcripts in this book, formal data analysis and manuscript preparation are yet to be done. It is possible that our attention will turn to Hispanic nurses or other racial or ethnocultural groups in the future, if we are able to locate collaborators.

None of my research would have been possible without the wonderful people who have collaborated with me on the various projects. I would like to name all of them for you now. Phase I team members were Kaye Bultemeier, Gayle Denham, Madge Donnellan, Patricia Droppleman, June Martin, Mary Anne Modrcin-McCarthy, Sheryl Russell, Pegge Saylor, Elizabeth Seabrook, Barbara Shirk, Carol Smucker, Jane Tollett, and Dorothy Wilt. The team that worked with me on the Phase II data were Janet Crooks, Janet Deese, Lucy Gasaway, Mary Pilkington, Donna Saravi, Patricia Droppleman, and Carol Smucker.

Team members for the African-American anger project were Becky Fields, Kelli Edwards, Angela Sims, Karen Reesman, Carolyn Robinson, Blair Short, and Belinda McCall. Contributors to the study of female nurses were Marilyn Smith, Patricia Droppleman, Janet Secrest, Linda Mefford, Tom McKay, and Phyllis Smith. Research group members at the time of the male nurses study were Aaron Brooks, Susan Blair, Lutie

Culver, Mitzi Davis, Jane Dozier, Patricia Droppleman, Phyllis duMont, Nancy Kile, Jerry Kline, Linda Mefford, Alicia Richardson, Marilyn Smith, Carol Smucker, and Susan Stuber. Howard Pollio's contribution to my understanding of phenomenology has been immeasurable, and I feel privileged to have participated in his weekly research group for the past 5 years. All of those five hundred or so pages of interview transcripts were typed by Linda Dalton, secretary for the University of Tennessee Center for Nursing Research. She has been an invaluable asset to all of our projects.

Finally, we must honor all of the courageous women and men who shared their work lives as nurses with us. Along with the rage and tears, there were many success stories of advocating for patients, using anger for self-empowerment, and lobbying for changes in ill-conceived institutional policies. I hope that these stories inspired you, as they did me. This program of research has been rewarding and enlightening to all of us on the investigative team. I know that the study participants will be pleased if you have benefited from what they shared with us.

References

Adams, B. L. (1997). Why must nurses risk their careers for safe care? *American Journal of Nursing, 97*(7), 80.

Acorn, S., Ratner, P., & Crawford, M. (1997). Decentralization as a determinant of autonomy, job satisfaction, and organizational commitment among nurse managers. *Nursing Research, 46,* 52–58.

Adkins, S. (1997). The privilege of intimacy. *Tennessee Nurse, 60*(2), 4.

Adler, A. (1956). *The individual psychology of Alfred Adler.* New York: Basic Books.

Adriaanse, H., Van Reek, J., Zandbelt, L., & Evers, G. (1991). Nurses' smoking worldwide: A review of 73 surveys on nurses' tobacco consumption in 21 countries in the period 1959–1988. *International Journal of Nursing Studies, 28*(4), 361–375.

Ahmadi, K. S., Speedling, E. J., & Kuhn-Weissman, G. (1987). The newly hired hospital staff nurse's professionalism, satisfaction and alienation. *International Journal of Nursing Studies, 24*(2), 107–121.

Aiken, L. (1992). Charting nursing's future. In L. Aiken & C. Fagin (Eds.), *Charting nursing's future: Agenda for the 1990s.* (pp. 3–12) Philadelphia: Lippincott.

Alberti, R., & Emmons, M. (1974). *Your perfect right: A guide to assertive behavior.* San Luis Obispo, CA: Impact Publishers.

Aldag, J., & Christensen, C. (1967). Personality correlates of male nurses. *Nursing Research, 16,* 375–376.

Aldwin, C., Sutton, K., & Lachman, M. (1996). The development of coping resources in adulthood. *Journal of Personality, 64,* 837–871.

American Nurses Association. (1993). *Sexual harassment: It's against the law.* Washington, DC: Author.

———. (1995). *Protect your patients, protect your license.* Washington, DC: Author.

———. (1996). *National survey reveals serious concerns among Americans about cost-cutting trends in patient care.* Washington, DC: Author.

American Nurses Publishing. (1993). *Nursing's agenda for health care reform.* Washington, DC: Author.

American Psychiatric Association. (1994). *Diagnostic and statistical manual of mental disorders,* (4th ed.). Washington, DC: Author.

Anderson, C. A. (1997). What is happening? *Nursing Outlook, 45,* 5–6.

Anderson, S. F., & Lawler, K. A. (1994, April). *Type A behavior in women and the anger recall interview: What are Type A women angry about and how do they express it?* Paper presented at the meeting of the Society of Behavioral Medicine, Boston.

Aneshensel, C. (1986). Marital and employment role-strain, social support, and depression among adult women. In S. Hobfoll (Ed.), *Stress, social support, and women* (pp. 99–114). Washington, DC: Hemisphere.

Angelou, M. (1993). *Wouldn't take nothing for my journey now.* New York: Random House.

Antonuccio, D. O., Danton, W. G., DeNelsky, G. Y. (1995). Psychotherapy versus medication for depression: Challenging the conventional wisdom with data. *Professional Psychology Research and Practice, 26,* 574–585.

Antonovsky, A. (1987). *Unraveling the mystery of health: How people manage stress and stay well.* San Francisco: Jossey-Bass.

Asher, R., & Hilton, I. (1996, September). *Security and investment in relationships: The impact on women's and men's anger.* Paper presented at the American Psychological Association Conference "Psychosocial and Behavioral Factors in Women's Health: Research, Prevention, Treatment, and Service Delivery in Clinical and Community Settings," Washington, DC.

Ashley, J. A. (1976). *Hospitals, paternalism, and the role of the nurse.* New York: Teachers College Press.

Ashley, M. J., Olin, J. S., Le-Riche, W., Kornaczewski, A., Schmidt, W., & Rankin, J. G. (1977). Morbidity in alcoholics: Evidence for accelerated development of physical disease in women. *Archives of Internal Medicine, 137,* 883–887.

Ausbrooks, E., Thomas, S. P., & Williams, R. (1995). Relationships among self-efficacy, optimism, trait anger, and anger expression. *Health Values, 19*(4), 46–53.

Averill, J. R. (1982). *Anger and aggression: An essay on emotion.* New York: Springer-Verlag.

———. (1983). Studies on anger and aggression: Implications for theories of emotion. *American Psychologist, 38,* 1145–1160.

Azar, B. (1997). Environment is key to serotonin levels. *American Psychological Association Monitor, 28*(4), 26, 29.

Babor, T. F., Lex, B. W., Mendelson, J. H., & Mello, N. K. (1984). Marijuana, effect and tolerance: A study of subchronic self-administration in women. In L. H. Harris (Ed.), *Problems of drug dependence (NIDA Research Monograph No. 49,* pp. 199–204). Washington, DC: U.S. Government Printing Office.

Bach, G., & Goldberg, H. (1974). *Creative aggression.* Garden City, NY: Anchor Books.

Barak, Y., Achiron, A., Kimh, R., Lampl, Y., Gilad, R., Elizur, A., & Sarova-Pinhas, I. (1996). Health risks among shift workers: A survey of female nurses. *Health Care for Women International, 17,* 527–533.

Barasch, M. (1993). *The healing path: A soul approach to illness.* New York: Penguin Books.

Barefoot, J. C., Peterson, B. L., Dahlstrom, W. G., Siegler, I. C., Anderson, N. B., & Williams, R. B. (1991). Hostility patterns and health implications: Correlates of Cook-Medley Hostility Scale scores in a national survey. *Health Psychology, 10,* 18–24.

Barnum, B. (1989). Anger and creating one's world. *Nursing and Health Care, 10*(5), 235.

Barritt, E. R. (1984). Inbreeding, infighting, and impotence. *American Journal of Nursing, 84,* 803–804.

Bass, B. M. (1997). Does the transactional-transformational leadership paradigm transcend organizational and national boundaries? *American Psychologist, 52,* 130–139.

Bateson, M. C. (1990). *Composing a life.* New York: Plume.

Baumeister, R. F., Stillwell, A., & Wotman, S. R. (1990). Victim and perpetrator accounts of interpersonal conflict: Autobiographical narratives about anger. *Journal of Personality and Social Psychology, 59,* 994–1005.

Beard, R. O. (1913). The trained nurse of the future. *Journal of the American Medical Association, 61,* 2149–2152.

Beaupre, P. M., Carney, R. M., Freedland, K. E., & Eisen, S. A. (1994, April). *The relation of depression and hostility to anginal symptoms and medication adherence in patients with coronary artery disease.* Paper presented at the meeting of the Society of Behavioral Medicine, Boston.

Beck, A. (1976). *Cognitive therapy and the emotional disorders.* New York: International Universities Press.

Beck, C. T. (1991). How students perceive faculty caring: A phenomenological study. *Nurse Educator, 16*(5), 18–22.

Bedell, J. R., & Lennox, S. S. (1996). *Handbook for communication and problem-solving skills training.* New York: Wiley.

Bell, R. (1984). Over-the-counter drugs: Factors in adult use of sedatives, tranquilizers, and stimulants. *Public Health Reports, 99,* 319–323.

Bennett, E. M. (1991). Weight loss practices of overweight adults. *American Journal of Clinical Nutrition, 53,* 1519S–1521S.

Benson, H. (1993). The relaxation response. In D. Goleman & J. Gurin (Eds.), *Mind/body medicine: How to use your mind for better health.* (pp. 233–257). Yonkers, NY: Consumer Reports Books.

Bernard, J. (1981). *The female world.* New York: Free Press.

Bernardez, T. (1987). Women and anger: Cultural prohibitions and the feminine ideal. *Work in progress: Stone Center for Developmental Services and Studies.* Wellesley, MA: Wellesley College, Stone Center.

Biaggio, M., & Godwin, W. (1987). Relation of depression to anger and hostility constructs. *Psychological Reports, 61,* 87–90.

Biener, L. (1987). Gender differences in the use of substances for coping. In R. C. Barnett, L. Biener, & G. K. Baruch (Eds.), *Gender and stress.* (pp. 330–349). New York: The Free Press.

Billings, A., & Moos, R. (1985). Psychosocial processes of remission in unipolar depression: Comparing depressed patients with matched community controls. *Journal of Consulting and Clinical Psychology, 53,* 314–325.

Birnbaum, D. W., & Croll, W. L. (1984). The etiology of children's stereotypes about sex differences in emotionality. *Sex Roles, 10,* 677–691.

Bishop, W. (1957). Florence Nightingale's letters. *American Journal of Nursing, 57,* 607–609.

Blegen, M. A. (1993). Nurses' job satisfaction: A meta-analysis of related variables. *Nursing Research, 42,* 36–41.

Block, J. (1973). Conceptions of sex role: Some cross-cultural and longitudinal perspectives. *American Psychologist, 28,* 512–526.

Block, K. (1997). The role of the self in healthy cancer survivorship: A view from the front lines of treating cancer. *Advances: The Journal of Mind-Body Health, 13*(1), 6–26.

Bohm, D. (1990). *On dialogue.* Ojai, CA: David Bohm Seminars.

Boltwood, M. D., Taylor, C. B., Burke, M. B., Grogin, H., & Giacomini, J. (1993). Anger report predicts coronary artery vasomotor response to mental stress in atherosclerotic segments. *American Journal of Cardiology, 72,* 1361–1365.

Bourke, D. H. (1997, May 17). Today's work has become hearth, altar. *St. Petersburg Times,* p. 8B.

Boyar, D. C., & Martinson, D. J. (1990). Intrapreneurial group practice. *Nursing and Health Care, 11*(1), 29–32.

Brandman, W. (1996). Intersubjectivity, social microcosm, and the here-and-now in a support group for nurses. *Archives of Psychiatric Nursing, 10,* 374–378.

Breda, K. L., Anderson, M. A., Hansen, L., Hayes, D., Pillion, C., & Lyon, P. (1997). Enhanced nursing autonomy through participatory action research. *Nursing Outlook, 45*(2), 76–81.

Briles, J. (1994). *The Briles report on women in health care.* San Francisco: Jossey-Bass.

Brody, J. (1994, September 5). Smoking halt tough for depression-prone. *The Knoxville News-Sentinel*, pp. B1, B2.

Brody, L. R. (1985). Gender differences in emotional development: A review of theories and research. *Journal of Personality, 53,* 102–149.

Bromberger, J. T., & Matthews, K. A. (1996). A "feminine" model of vulnerability to depressive symptoms: A longitudinal investigation of middle-aged women. *Journal of Personality and Social Psychology, 70*(3), 591–598.

Brondolo, E. (1992, March). *Confiding versus confronting: Gender differences in anger expression among children and adolescents.* Paper presented at the meeting of the Society of Behavioral Medicine, New York.

Brondolo, E., Bendetto, M., Storrs, J., Baruch, C., & Contrada, R. (1993, March). *The effects of conflict management style on ambulatory blood pressure among NYC traffic agents.* Paper presented at the meeting of the Society of Behavioral Medicine, San Francisco.

Brookfield, G., Douglas, A., Shapiro, R., & Cias, S. (1988). Some thoughts on being a male in nursing. In J. Muff (Ed.), *Socialization, sexism, and stereotyping: Women's issues in nursing* (pp. 273–277). Prospect Heights, IL: Waveland Press.

Brooks, A., Thomas, S. P., & Droppleman, P. (1996). From frustration to red fury: A description of work-related anger in male registered nurses. *Nursing Forum, 31*(3), 4–15.

Brown, L., & Gilligan, C. (1992). *Meeting at the crossroads: Women's psychology and girls' development.* Cambridge, MA: Harvard University Press.

Browne, A., & Finkelhor, D. (1986). Impact of child sexual abuse: A review of the research. *Psychological Bulletin, 99*(1), 66–77.

Browning, L. (1994). Government affairs. *Tennessee Nurse, 57*(1), 9.

Buber, M. (1965). *Between man and man.* New York: Macmillan.

Bullough, V. L. (1990). Nightingale, nursing and harassment. *Image: Journal of Nursing Scholarship, 22*(1), 4–7.

Bullough, V. L., Church, O. M., & Stein, A. (1988). *American nursing: A biographical dictionary.* New York: Garland.

Buresh, B., & Gordon, S. (1996). Subtle self-sabotage. *American Journal of Nursing, 96*(4), 22–24.

Burns, J. M. (1978). *Leadership.* New York: Harper & Row.

Bush, J. (1988). Job satisfaction, powerlessness, and locus of control. *Western Journal of Nursing Research, 10,* 718–731.

Cafferata, G., Kasper, J., & Bernstein, A. (1983). Family roles, structure, and stressors in relation to sex differences in obtaining psychotropic drugs. *Journal of Health and Social Behavior, 24,* 132–143.

Cahill, S. (1997, March 3). The Wal-Mart of hospitals. *In These Times*, pp. 14–16.

Campbell, A. (1984). Nursing, nurturing, and sexism. In A. Campbell (Ed.), *Moderated love: A theology of professional care* (pp. 34–51). London: SPCK.

Campbell, A. (1993). *Men, women, and aggression.* New York: Basic Books.

Canavan, K. (1997a). Media embraces ANA's concerns about unsafe patient care. *The American Nurse, 29*(3), 1, 12.

———. (1997b). Combating dangerous delegation. *American Journal of Nursing, 97*(5), 57–58.

———. (1997c). Nurses confront whistle-blower retaliations. *The American Nurse, 29*(3), 12.

———. (1997d). ANA study links nurse staffing to quality. *The American Nurse, 29*(3), 1,3.

Carlson-Catalano, J. (1990). Hospital nurse experiences. In L. Gasparis & J. Swirsky (Eds.), *Nurse abuse: Its impact and resolution* (pp. 125–174). New York: Power Publications.

Carmack, B. J. (1997). Balancing engagement and detachment in caregiving. *Image: Journal of Nursing Scholarship, 29,* 139–143.

Caroline, H., & Bernhard, L. (1994). Health care dilemmas for women with serious mental illness. *Advances in Nursing Science, 16*(3), 78–88.

Carroll, J. (1993, July 1). The first baby can put a marriage under a lot of stress. *The Knoxville News-Sentinel,* p. B3.

Cautela, J. (1969). Behavior therapy and self-control: Techniques and implications. In C. M. Franks (Ed.), *Behavior therapy: Appraisal and status* (pp. 323–340). New York: McGraw-Hill.

Chernin, K. (1985). *The hungry self: Women, eating, and identity.* New York: Harper & Row.

Cherniss, C. (1995). *Beyond burnout: Helping teachers, nurses, therapists, and lawyers recover from stress and disillusionment.* New York: Routledge.

Chinn, P. L. (1991). Looking into the crystal ball: Positioning ourselves for the year 2000. *Nursing Outlook, 39,* 251–256.

Christen, A. G., & Cooper, K. H. (1979). *Strategic withdrawal from cigarette smoking.* New York: American Cancer Society.

Christman, L. (1988). Luther Christman. In T. Schorr & A. Zimmerman (Eds.), *Making choices, taking chances: Nurse leaders tell their stories* (pp. 43–52). St. Louis: Mosby.

Church, G. J. (1997). Backlash against HMOs. *Time, 149*(15), 32–36.

Cleary, D. M. (1975). A nonstrike for patient care. *Modern Healthcare, 3*(6), 43–44.

Colgrove, M., Bloomfield, H., & McWilliams, P. (1991). *How to survive the loss of a love.* Los Angeles: Prelude Press. (Original work published 1976)

Constable, J., & Russell, D. (1986). The effect of social support and the work environment upon burnout among nurses. *Journal of Human Stress, 12*(1), 20–26.

Cook, E. (1913). *The life of Florence Nightingale.* London: Macmillan.

Cooper, S. S. (1997). Men who choose nursing. *Nursing Dimensions, 8,* 24–26.

Cooperstock, R. (1978). Sex differences in psychotropic drug use. *Social Science and Medicine, 12B,* 179–186.

Copp, L. A. (1995). Dean-bashing. *Journal of Professional Nursing, 11*(1), 1–2.

Cox, H. (1991, January). Verbal abuse nationwide: Part 1. Oppressed group behavior. *Nursing Management, 22,* 32–35.

Crawford, J., Kippax, S., Onyx, J., Gault, U., & Benton, P. (1990). Women theorizing their experiences of anger: A study using memory-work. *Australian Psychologist, 25,* 333–350.

Cronin-Stubbs, D., & Velsor-Friedrich, B. (1981). Professional and personal stress: A survey. *Nursing Leadership, 4,* 19.

Crouch, M. A., & Straub, V. (1983). Enhancement of self-esteem in adults. *Family and Community Health, 6*(2), 65–78.

Crownover, A. (1995, November 29). Don't replace RNs with unlicensed assistive personnel. *Nashville Banner.*

Cummings, N. (1996). Now we're facing the consequences. *The Scientist Practitioner, 6*(1), 9–13.

Cummings, S. H. (1995). Attila the Hun versus Attila the hen: Gender socialization of the American nurse. *Nursing Administration Quarterly, 19*(2), 19–29.

Curtin, L. (1995). To see ourselves. . . . *Nursing Management, 26*(9), 7–8.

Dafter, R. E. (1996). Why "negative" emotions can sometimes be positive: The spectrum model of emotions and their role in mind-body healing. *Advances: The Journal of Mind-Body Health, 12*(2), 6–19.

Daley, K. A. (1997). The power of unity. *American Journal of Nursing, 97*(3), 80.

Dattilo, A. M., & Kris-Etherton, P. M. (1992). Effects of weight reduction on blood lipids and lipoproteins: A meta-analysis. *American Journal of Clinical Nutrition, 56,* 320–328.

Davidson, D. (1987). Every nurse an OR manager: How well does it work? *OR Manager, 3*(3), 3.

Davies, C. (1995). *Gender and the professional predicament in nursing.* Philadelphia: Open University Press.

DeAngelis, T. (1997). When children don't bond with parents. *American Psychological Association Monitor, 28*(6), 10, 12.

Deffenbacher, J. (1992). Trait anger: Theory, findings, and implications. In C. D. Spielberger & J. N. Butcher (Eds.), *Advances in personality assessment* (Vol. 9, pp. 177–201). Hillsdale, NJ: Erlbaum.

———. (1994, August). *Anger does not equal aggression.* Paper presented at the meeting of the American Psychological Association, Los Angeles.

————. (1995a, August). *Assessing forms of anger expression.* Paper presented at the meeting of the American Psychological Association, New York.

————. (1995b). Ideal treatment package for adults with anger disorders. In H. Kassinove (Ed.), *Anger disorders: Definition, diagnosis, and treatment* (pp. 151–172). Washington, DC: Taylor & Francis.

Deffenbacher, J., Oetting, E., Lynch, R., & Morris, C. (1996). The expression of anger and its consequences. *Behaviour Research and Therapy, 34,* 575–590.

Derogatis, L., Abeloff, M., & Melisaratos, N. (1979). Psychological coping mechanisms and survival time in metastatic breast cancer. *Journal of the American Medical Association, 242,* 1504–1508.

Diaz, A. L., & McMillin, J. D. (1991). A definition and description of nurse abuse. *Western Journal of Nursing Research, 13*(1), 97–109.

Dixon, J. P., Dixon, J. K., & Spinner, J. C. (1991). Tensions between career and interpersonal commitments as a risk factor for cardiovascular disease among women. *Women and Health, 17*(3), 33–57.

Doherty, R., Orimoto, L., Singelis, T., Hatfield, E., & Hebb, J. (1995). Emotional contagion: Gender and occupational differences. *Psychology of Women Quarterly, 19,* 355–371.

Donahue, M. P. (1985). *Nursing: The finest art.* St. Louis: Mosby.

Dossey, B. (1995). Nurse as healer. In B. Dossey, L. Keegan, C. Guzzetta, & L. Kolkmeier (Eds.), *Holistic nursing: A handbook for practice* (2nd ed., pp. 61–82). Gaithersburg, MD: Aspen.

Dossey, L. (1984). *Beyond illness.* Boston: Shambhala Publications.

Droppleman, P., & Wilt, D. (1993). Women, depression, and anger. In S. P. Thomas (Ed.), *Women and anger* (pp. 209–232). New York: Springer.

Dryden, W. (1990). *Dealing with anger problems: Rational-emotive therapeutic interventions.* Sarasota, FL: Professional Resource Exchange.

Duquette, A., Kerouac, S., Sandhu, B., & Beaudet, L. (1994). Factors related to nursing burnout: A review of empirical knowledge. *Issues in Mental Health Nursing, 15,* 337–358.

Durel, L. A., Carver, C. S., Spitzer, S. B., Llabre, M. M., Weintraub, J. K., Saab, P. G., & Schneiderman, N. (1989). Associations of blood pressure with self-report measures of anger and hostility among black and white men and women. *Health Psychology, 8,* 557–575.

Eagly, A., & Steffen, V. (1986). Gender and aggressive behavior: A meta-analytic review of the social psychological literature. *Psychological Bulletin, 100,* 309–330.

Eisenstein, H. (1988). On the psychosocial barriers to professions for women. In J. Muff (Ed.), *Women's issues in nursing: Socialization, sexism, and stereotyping.* (pp. 95–112). Prospect Heights, IL: Waveland Press.

Ekman, P. (1994). All emotions are basic. In P. Ekman & R. J. Davidson (Eds.), *The nature of emotion: Fundamental questions* (pp. 15–19). New York: Oxford University Press.

Elkind, A. K. (1988). Do nurses smoke because of stress? *Journal of Advanced Nursing, 13,* 733–745.

Ellis, A. (1973). *Humanistic psychotherapy: The rational-emotive approach.* New York: The Julian Press.

Ellis, L. (1980). An investigation of nursing student self-concept levels: A pilot study. *Nursing Research, 29,* 389–390.

Emerson, C., & Harrison, D. (1990). Anger and denial as predictors of cardiovascular reactivity in women. *Journal of Psychopathology and Behavioral Assessment, 12,* 271–283.

Engebretson, T. O., Matthews, K. A., & Scheier, M. F. (1989). Relations between anger expression and cardiovascular reactivity: Reconciling inconsistent findings through a matching hypothesis. *Journal of Personality and Social Psychology, 57,* 513–521.

Epstein, A. H. (1989). *Mind, fantasy and healing: One woman's journey from conflict and illness to wholeness and health.* New York: Delacorte Press.

Erlen, J., & Frost, B. (1991). Nurses' perceptions of powerlessness in influencing ethical decisions. *Western Journal of Nursing Research, 13,* 397–407.

Evans, D. R., Hearn, M. T., & Saklofske, D. (1973). Anger, arousal, and systematic desensitization. *Psychological Reports, 32,* 625–626.

Evans, P. D., & Edgerton, N. (1991). Life-events and mood as predictors of the common cold. *British Journal of Medical Psychology, 64*(1), 35–44.

Ewart, C. K., Taylor, C. B., Kraemer, H. C., & Agras, W. S. (1991). High blood pressure and marital discord: Not being nasty matters more than being nice. *Health Psychology, 10,* 155–163.

Ewashen, C. J. (1997). Devaluation dynamics and gender bias in women's groups. *Issues in Mental Health Nursing, 18,* 73–84.

Extended Services Team, Visiting Nurse Association of Northern Virginia. (1997). Wellness for nurses, by nurses. *American Journal of Nursing, 97*(5), 67–68.

Fagin, C. (1994). Women and nursing, today and tomorrow. In E. Friedman (Ed.), *An unfinished revolution: Women and health care in America* (pp. 159–176). New York: United Hospital Fund of New York.

Fagot, B. I., Leinbach, M. D., & Hagan, R. (1986). Gender labeling and the development of sex-typed behaviors. *Developmental Psychology, 22,* 440–443.

Feindler, E. L., & Ecton, R. B. (1986). *Adolescent anger control: Cognitive-behavioral techniques.* New York: Pergamon Press.

Ferguson, P., & Small, W. P. (1985). Further study of the smoking habits of hospital nurses. *Health Bulletin, 43*(1), 13–18.

Fiore, M. C., Novotny, T. E., Pierce, J. P., Giovino, G., Hatziandreau, E. J., Newcomb, P., Surawicz, T., & Davis, R. (1990). Methods used to quit smoking in the United States: Do cessation programs help? *Journal of the American Medical Association, 263,* 2760–2765.

Firth, H., McKeown, P., McIntee, J., & Britton, P. (1987). Professional depression, "burnout" and personality in longstay nursing. *International Journal of Nursing Studies, 24,* 227–237.

Fiske, S. T. (1993). Controlling other people: The impact of power on stereotyping. *American Psychologist, 48,* 621–628.

Fitzgerald, L. (1993). Sexual harassment: Violence against women in the workplace. *American Psychologist, 48,* 1070–1076.

Fleming, M. F., & Barry, K. L. (1992). *Addictive disorders.* St. Louis: Mosby.

Folkman, S., & Lazarus, R. (1980). Stress processes and depressive symptomatology. *Journal of Abnormal Psychology, 95,*107–113.

Fondiller, S. H. (1995). Loretta C. Ford: A modern Olympian. *Nursing and Health Care: Perspectives on Community, 16*(1), 6–11.

Forest, K. B. (1991). The interplay of childhood stress and adult life events on women's symptoms of depression. *Dissertation Abstracts International, 51*(9A), 3237.

Forster, J. L., & Jeffery, R. W. (1986). Gender differences related to weight history, eating patterns, efficacy expectations, self-esteem, and weight loss among participants in a weight reduction program. *Addictive Behaviors, 11,* 141–147.

Fowler, C. M. (1996). *Before women had wings.* New York: Fawcett Columbine.

Frankl, V. (1978). *The unheard cry for meaning.* New York: Simon & Schuster.

Freiberg, P. (1991). Self-esteem gender gap widens in adolescence. *American Psychological Association Monitor, 22*(4), 29.

Frey, W., & Langseth, M. (1985). *Crying: The mystery of tears.* Minneapolis: Winston.

Frezza, M., DiPadova, C., Pozzato, G., Terpin, M., Baraona, E., & Lieber, C. (1990). High blood alcohol levels in women: The role of decreased gastric alcohol dehydrogenase and first-pass metabolism. *New England Journal of Medicine, 322*(2), 95–99.

Friedman, A. S. (1970). Hostility factors and clinical improvement in depressed patients. *Archives of General Psychiatry, 23,* 524–537.

Friedman, M., & Rosenman, R. (1974) *Type A behavior and your heart.* New York: Knopf.

Future of nursing scholarship. (1997). *Image: Journal of Nursing Scholarship, 29,* 117–121.

Gallop, R., McKeever, P., Toner, B., Lancee, W., & Lueck, M. (1995). The impact of childhood sexual abuse on the psychological well-being and practice of nurses. *Archives of Psychiatric Nursing, 9*(3), 137–145.

Garmezy, N., & Neuchterlain, K. (1972). Invulnerable children: The fact and fiction of competence and disadvantage. *American Journal of Orthopsychiatry, 42,* 328–329.

Garant, F. (1981). Power, leadership, and nursing. *Nursing Forum, 20,* 183–199.

Gaskin, J. (1986). Nurses in trouble. *Canadian Nurse, 82*(4), 31–34.

Gauvin, L., Rejeski, W. J., & Norris, J. L. (1996). *Health Psychology, 15,* 391–397.

Gendlin, E. (1973). A phenomenology of emotions: Anger. In D. Carr & E. S. Casey (Eds.), *Explorations in phenomenology* (pp. 367–398). The Hague, Netherlands: Martinus Nijhoff.

George, T. (1997, June). *Mono-sexual tradition in philosophy, epistemology, and the work world of women.* Paper presented at the Eighth International Congress on Women's Health Issues, Saskatoon, Saskatchewan.

Gerlock, A. A. (1994). Veterans' responses to anger management intervention. *Issues in Mental Health Nursing, 15,* 393–408.

Gianakos, D. (1997). Physicians, nurses, and collegiality. *Nursing Outlook, 45*(2), 57–58.

Ginzberg, E. (1997). Managed care and the competitive market in health care: What they can and cannot do. *Journal of the American Medical Association, 277*(22), 1812–1813.

Ginzberg, E., & Ostow, M. (1997). Managed care: A look back and a look ahead. *The New England Journal of Medicine, 336*(14), 1018–1020.

Godwin, G. (1983). *Mr. Bedford and the Muses.* New York: Ballantine.

Goertzel, V., & Goertzel, M. G. (1962). *Cradles of eminence.* Boston: Little, Brown.

Goffman, E. (1967). *Interaction ritual.* Garden City, NY: Doubleday.

Goldstein, D. J. (1991). Beneficial health effects of modest weight loss. *International Journal of Obesity, 16,* 397–415.

Goleman, D. (1995). *Emotional intelligence.* New York: Bantam.

Goodman, M., Quigley, J., Moran, G., Meilman, H., & Sherman, M. (1996). Hostility predicts restenosis after percutaneous transluminal coronary angioplasty. *Mayo Clinic Proceedings, 71,* 729–734.

Gorman, M. (1997). Helping patients to quit smoking. *American Journal of Nursing, 97*(3), 64–65.

Gorman, S., & Clark, N. (1986). Power and effective nursing practice. *Nursing Outlook, 34,* 129–134.

Greer, G. (1991). *The change.* New York: Fawcett Columbine.

Greer, S., & Morris, T. (1975). Psychological attitudes of women who develop breast cancer: A controlled study. *Journal of Psychosomatic Research, 19,* 147–153.

Greer, S., Morris, T., Pettingale, K. W., & Haybittle, J. L. (1990). Psychological response to breast cancer and fifteen-year outcome. *Lancet, 335*(1), 49–50.

Greif, E., Alvarez, M., & Ulman, L. (1981, April). *Recognizing emotions in other people: Sex differences in socialization.* Paper presented at the biennial meeting of the Society for Research in Child Development, Boston.

Grilo, C. M., Shiffman, S., & Wing, R. (1989). Relapse crises and coping among dieters. *Journal of Consulting and Clinical Psychology, 57,* 488–495.

Gropper, E. (1994). Women supporting women: Are nurses really their own worst enemies? *Nursing Forum, 29*(3), 34–36.

Grossarth-Maticek, R., Bastiaans, J., & Kanazir, D. (1985). Psychosocial factors as strong predictors of mortality from cancer, ischemic heart disease and stroke: The Yugoslav prospective study. *Journal of Psychosomatic Research, 29,* 167–176.

Grothgar, B., & Scholz, D. B. (1987). On specific behavior of migraine patients in an anger provoking situation. *Headache, 27,* 206–210.

Grover, S. M., & Thomas, S. P. (1993). Substance use and anger in midlife women. *Issues in Mental Health Nursing, 14,* 19–29.

Groves, J. (1978). Taking care of the hateful patient. *New England Journal of Medicine, 298,* 883–887.

Gulack, R. (1983, December). Why nurses leave nursing. *RN, 46,* 32–37.

Gut, E. (1989). *Productive and unproductive depression.* New York: Basic Books.

Gutierrez, L. (1990, March). Working with women of color: An empowerment perspective. *Social Work,* pp. 149–153.

Hagberg, J. (1984). *Real power.* Minneapolis: Winston.

Hall, S. S. (1989, June). A molecular code links emotions, mind and health. *Smithsonian,* pp. 62–70.

Halsey, J. (1985, Winter). The moderately troubled nurse: A not-so-uncommon entity. *Nursing Administration Quarterly,* 69–76.

Harburg, E., Blakelock, E., & Roeper, P. (1979). Resentful and reflective coping with arbitrary authority and blood pressure: Detroit. *Psychosomatic Medicine, 41,* 189–199.

Hart, P. D. (1990). *A nation-wide survey of attitudes towards health care and nurses.* Washington, DC: Hart Research Associates.

Hart, S. (1997). A gift disguised. *American Journal of Nursing, 97*(6), 54.

Hastings, C., & Waltz, C. (1995). Assessing the outcome of professional practice redesign: Impact on staff nurse perceptions. *Journal of Nursing Administration, 25*(3), 34–42.

Haynes, S., & Feinleib, M. (1980). Women, work and coronary heart disease: Prospective findings from the Framingham Heart Study. *American Journal of Public Health, 70,* 133–141.

Haynes, S., Feinleib, M., & Kannel, W. (1980). The relationship of psychosocial factors to coronary heart disease in the Framingham Study. *American Journal of Epidemiology, 111,* 37–58.

Haynes, S., Feinleib, M., Levine, S., Scotch, N., & Kannel, W. (1978). The relationship of psychosocial factors to coronary heart disease in the Framingham Study: II. Prevalence of coronary heart disease. *American Journal of Epidemiology, 107,* 384–402.

Haynes, S., Levine, S., Scotch, N., Feinleib, M., & Kannel, W. (1978). The relationship of psychosocial factors to coronary heart disease in the Framingham Study: I. Methods and risk factors. *American Journal of Epidemiology, 107,* 362–383.

Hazaleus, S., & Deffenbacher, J. (1985, January). Irrational beliefs and anger arousal. *Journal of College Student Personnel,* pp. 47–52.

Hazaleus, S., & Deffenbacher, J. (1986). Relaxation and cognitive treatments of anger. *Journal of Consulting and Clinical Psychology, 54,* 222–226.

Hearn, M. T., & Evans, D. R. (1972). Anger and reciprocal inhibition therapy. *Psychological Reports, 30,* 943–948.

Hecker, M., Chesney, M., Black, G., & Frautschi, N. (1989). Coronary-prone behaviors in the Western Collaborative Group Study. *Psychosomatic Medicine, 50,* 153–164.

Hedin, A. (1994). *Perceived total workload stress, stress symptoms and coping styles of working women.* Unpublished doctoral dissertation. University of Maryland, College Park.

Heide, W. (1988). Feminist activism in nursing and health care. In J. Muff (Ed.), *Women's issues in nursing: Socialization, sexism, and stereotyping* (pp. 255–272). Prospect Heights, IL: Waveland Press.

Heim, P. (1995). Getting beyond "she said, he said." *Nursing Administration Quarterly, 19*(2), 6–18.

Hellman, L. (1973). *Pentimento.* Boston: Little, Brown.

Helmlinger, C. (1997). A growing physical workload threatens nurses' health. *American Journal of Nursing, 97*(4), 64–66.

Henley, N. (1977). *Body politics: Power, sex, and nonverbal communication.* Englewood Cliffs, NJ: Prentice-Hall.

Herman, S. (1978). *Becoming assertive: A guide for nurses.* New York: Van Nostrand.

Hillhouse, J., & Adler, C. (1997). Investigating stress effect patterns in hospital staff nurses: Results of a cluster analysis. *Social Science and Medicine, 45,* 1781–1788.

Hochschild, A. R. (1979). Emotion work, feeling rules, and social structure. *American Journal of Sociology, 85,* 551–575.

Hochschild, A. R. (1997). *The time bind: When work becomes home and home becomes work.* New York: Henry Holt.

Hollis, J. (1994). *Fat and furious: Women and food obsession.* New York: Fawcett.

Holz, K. (1994). A practical approach to clients who are survivors of childhood sexual abuse. *Journal of Nurse Midwifery, 39*(1), 13–18.

Horton, J. A. (Ed.). (1992). *The women's health data book.* Washington, DC: Jacobs Institute of Women's Health.

Hughes, J. R. (1985). *The relationship between smoking and mood: Role of smoking in affect regulation.* Symposium presented at the meeting of the Society of Behavioral Medicine, New Orleans.

Hutchinson, S. (1986). Chemically dependent nurses: The trajectory toward self-annihilation. *Nursing Research, 35,* 196–201.

Institute for Health and Socio-Economic Policy. (1996). Wealth and power: The U.S. Health Care Industry. *Revolution: The Journal of Nurse Empowerment, 6*(4), 67–70.

Ironson, G., Taylor, C. B., Boltwood, M., Bartzokis, T., Dennis, C., Chesney, M., Spitzer, S., & Segall, G. (1992). Effects of anger on left ventricular ejection fraction in coronary artery disease. *American Journal of Cardiology, 70,* 281–285.

Isler, C. (1970). Florence Nightingale: The call to war, *RN, 33* (5), 42–45, 74.

Jacklin, C., & Maccoby, E. (1978). Social behavior at 33 months in same-sex and mixed-sex dyads. *Child Development, 49,* 557–569.

Jacobson, S. F. (1983). An overview of coping. In S. F. Jacobson & H. M. McGrath (Eds.), *Nurses under stress.* (pp. 26–46). New York: Wiley.

Jacobson, S., & McGrath, H. M. (Eds.). *Nurses under stress.* New York: Wiley.

Jarratt, V. (1981, July). Why do nurses eat their young? *The Arkansas State Nursing Association Newsletter, 1*(2), 4, 10.

Jenkins, J. (1996). Nursing in the new millennium. *Tennessee Nurse, 59*(2), 17–19.

Jones, J. W. (1982). *The burnout syndrome.* New York: London House.

Josefowitz, N. (1980). *Paths to power: A woman's guide from first job to top executive.* Reading, MA: Addison Wesley.

Jourard, S. (1971). *The transparent self.* New York: Van Nostrand.

Julius, M., Harburg, E., Schork, M., & DiFrancisco, W. (1992, March). *Differential impact of suppressed anger on cardiovascular and cancer mortality for married pairs (Tecumseh 1971–1988).* Paper presented at the meeting of the Society of Behavioral Medicine, New York.

Jung, C. G. (1965). *Memories, dreams, reflections.* New York: Vintage.

Kabb, G. (1984). Chemical dependency: Helping your staff. *Journal of Nursing Administration, 14*(11), 18–23.

Kagan, D. M., & Squires, R. L. (1984). Compulsive eating, dieting, stress, and hostility among college students. *Journal of College Student Personnel, 25,* 213–220.

Kalisch, B. J., & Kalisch, P. A. (1975). Slaves, servants, or saints? An analysis of the system of nurse training in the United States, 1873–1948. *Nursing Forum, 14,* 222–263.

———. (1977). An analysis of the sources of physician-nurse conflict. *Journal of Nursing Administration, 7*(1), 51–57.

Kanter, R. M. (1977). *Men and women of the corporation.* New York: Basic Books.

Kaplan, D. (1997). When less is more. *Psychology Today, 30*(3), 14.

Kawachi, I., Sparrow, D., Spiro, A., Vokonas, P., & Weiss, S. (1996). A prospective study of anger and coronary heart disease: The Normative Aging Study. *Circulation, 94,* 2090–2095.

Keddy, B. C. (1995). Feminist teaching and the older nurse: The journey from resistance through anger to hope. *Journal of Advanced Nursing, 21,* 690–694.

Keepin, W. (1994, Summer). David Bohm: A life of dialogue between science and spirit. *Noetic Sciences Review* pp. 10–16.

Kelley, J. (1997, May 5). Swiss nurse independently saved Nazis' youngest targets. *USA Today,* p. 2D.

Kesey, K. (1973). *One flew over the cuckoo's nest.* New York: Picador.

Kilbey, M., & Sobeck, J. (1988). Epidemiology of alcoholism. In C. B. Travis (Ed.), *Women and health psychology: Mental health issues* (pp. 91–107). Hillsdale, NJ: Erlbaum.

Kitson, A. L. (1997). Johns Hopkins address: Does nursing have a future? *Image: Journal of Nursing Scholarship, 29,* 111–115.

Kleehammer, K., Hart, A. L., & Keck, J. F. (1990). Nursing students' perceptions of anxiety-producing situations in the clinical setting. *Journal of Nursing Education, 29,* 183–187.

Knaus, W. A., Draper, E. A., Wagner, D. P., & Zimmerman, J. E. (1986). An evaluation of outcome from intensive care in major medical centers. *Annals of Internal Medicine, 104,* 410–418.

Kolkmeier, L. G. (1995). Relaxation: Opening the door to change. In B. M. Dossey, L. Keegan, C. E. Guzzetta, & L. G. Kolkmeier (Eds.), *Holistic nursing: A handbook for practice* (pp. 573–605). Gaithersburg, MD: Aspen.

Kollar, M., Groer, M., Thomas, S., & Cunningham, J. (1991). Adolescent anger: A developmental study. *Journal of Child and Adolescent Psychiatric Nursing, 4,* 9–15.

Kopper, B., & Epperson, D. (1991). Women and anger: Sex and sex-role comparisons in the expression of anger. *Psychology of Women Quarterly, 15,* 7–14.

Kornfield, J. (1993). *A path with heart.* New York: Bantam.

Kraegel, J., & Kachoyeanos, M. (1989). *Just a nurse.* New York: Dell.

Kramer, M. (1974). *Reality shock.* St. Louis: Mosby.

Krucoff, C. (1997, May 6). Man's best exercise buddy: Secrets I've learned from my four-legged partner. *The Washington Post, Health,* p. 20.

Kune, G., Kune, S., Watson, L., & Bahnson, C. (1991). Personality as a risk factor in large bowel cancer: Data from the Melbourne Colorectal Cancer Study. *Psychological Medicine, 21,* 28–41.

Kunen, J. (1996, September 30). The new hands-off nursing. *Time,* pp. 56–57.

Lancee, W. J., Gallop, R., McCay, E., & Toner, B. (1995). The relationship between nurses' limit-setting styles and anger in psychiatric inpatients. *Psychiatric Services, 46*(6), 609–613.

Lanza, M. L. (1983). The reactions of nursing staff to physical assault by a patient. *Hospital and Community Psychiatry, 34,* 44–47.

Lanza, M. L., Kayne, H. L., Pattison, I., Hicks, C., & Islam, S. (1996). The relationship of behavioral cues to assaultive behavior. *Clinical Nursing Research, 5*(1), 6–27.

Larson, D. G. (1987). Helper secrets: Internal stressors in nursing. *Journal of Psychosocial Nursing and Mental Health Services, 25*(4), 20–27.

Larson, E. L. (1995). New rules for the game: Interdisciplinary education for health professionals. *Nursing Outlook, 43,* 180–185.

Lazarus, R. S. (1991). *Emotion and adaptation.* New York: Oxford University Press.

Leach, R. A. (1990, September 6). Anecdote about butterfly's wings cures the blahs. *Nashville Banner,* p. A15.

Lemaire, T., & Clopton, J. (1981). Expressions of hostility in mild depression. *Psychological Reports, 48,* 259–262.

Lerner, H. G. (1985). *The dance of anger: A woman's guide to changing the patterns of intimate relationships.* New York: Harper & Row.

Lerner, M. J. (1980). *The belief in a just world: A fundamental delusion.* New York: Plenum.

Lever, J. (1976). Sex differences in the games children play. *Social Problems, 23,* 478–487.

Levey, G. A. (1994, November 13). What's your mood food? *Parade Magazine,* p. 16.

Levine, M. E. (1970). The intransigent patient. *American Journal of Nursing, 70,* 2106–2111.

Levinson, D. J. (1978). *The seasons of a man's life.* New York: Knopf.

———. (1996). *The seasons of a woman's life.* New York: Ballantine.

Levinson, H. (1980). Power, leadership, and the management of stress. *Professional Psychology, 11,* 497–508.

Lex, B. W. (1991). Some gender differences in alcohol and polysubstance users. *Health Psychology, 10,* 121–132.

Lexicon Publications. (1989). *The New Lexicon Webster's Dictionary of the English Language.* New York: Author.

Libbus, M. K., & Bowman, K. G. (1997, June). *Sexual harassment: Development of an instrument to assess staff nurse sensitivity.* Paper presented at the Eighth International Congress on Women's Health Issues, Saskatoon, Saskatchewan.

Little, M. (1991). America's secret. *Tennessee Nurse, 54*(6), 16–19.

―――. (1993). AMA's new smear campaign—fowl play. *Tennessee Nurse, 56*(4), 12–14.

Lovell, M. C. (1988). Daddy's little girl: The lethal effects of paternalism in nursing. In J. Muff (Ed.), *Women's issues in nursing: Socialization, sexism and stereotyping* (pp. 210–220). Prospect Heights, IL: Waveland Press.

Lucas, M. D., Atwood, J. R., & Hagaman, R. (1993). Replication and validation of anticipated turnover model for urban registered nurses. *Nursing Research, 42,* 29–35.

Macnee, C. (1991). Perceived well-being of persons quitting smoking. *Nursing Research, 40,* 200–203.

Mainiero, L. A. (1986). Coping with powerlessness: The relationship of gender and job dependency to empowerment-strategy usage. *Administrative Science Quarterly, 31,* 633–653.

Malone, B. (1985, Winter). Legitimate anger: Consequences and challenges. *Nursing Administration Quarterly,* 41–45.

Manderino, M. A., & Berkey, N. (1995). Verbal abuse of staff nurses by physicians. *Image: Journal of Nursing Scholarship, 27*(3), 244.

Mansen, T. J. (1993). Role-taking abilities of nursing education administrators and their perceived leadership effectiveness. *Journal of Professional Nursing, 9,* 347–357.

Marks, S. (1979, Summer). Culture, human energy, and self-actualization: A sociological offering to humanistic psychology. *Journal of Humanistic Psychology, 19*(3), 27–42.

Marszalek-Gaucher, E., & Elsenhans, V. (1988). Intrapreneurship: Tapping employee creativity. *Journal of Nursing Administration, 18*(12), 20–22.

Maslach, C. (1982). *Burnout: The cost of caring.* Englewood Cliffs, NJ: Prentice-Hall.

Mason, R. (1995). PACDN update: The Peer Assistance for Chemically Dependent Nurses (PACDN) Committee. *Virginia Nurses Today, 3*(3), 15–17.

McGrath, E., Keita, G., Strickland, B., & Russo, N. (1990). *Women and depression: Risk factors and treatment issues.* Washington, DC: American Psychological Association.

McWilliams, N., & Stein, J. (1987). Women's groups led by women: The management of devaluing transferences. *International Journal of Group Psychotherapy, 37,* 139–153.

Meissner, J. (1986). Nurses: Are we eating our young? *Nursing, 16*(3), 51–53.

Merleau-Ponty, M. (1962). *The phenomenology of perception.* London: Routledge & Kegan Paul.

Miller, J. B. (1983). The construction of anger in men and women. *Work in progress: Stone Center for Developmental Services and Studies.* Wellesley, MA: Wellesley College, Stone Center.

Minnick, A., Roberts, M., Young, W., Marcantonio, R., & Kleinpell, R. (1997). Ethnic diversity and staff nurse employment in hospitals. *Nursing Outlook, 45*(1), 35–40.

Mittleman, M. A., Maclure, M., Sherwood, J. B., Mulry, R. P., Tofler, G. H., Jacobs, S. C., Friedman, R., Benson, H., & Muller, J. E. (1995). Triggering of acute myocardial infarction onset by episodes of anger. *Circulation, 92*(1), 720–725.

Monteiro, L. (1985). Florence Nightingale on public health nursing. *American Journal of Public Health, 75,* 181–186.

Montgomery, C. L. (1991). The care-giving relationship: Paradoxical and transcendent aspects. *Journal of Transpersonal Psychology, 13*(2), 91–104.

Moon, J. R., & Eisler, R. M. (1983). Anger control: An experimental comparison of three behavioral treatments. *Behavior Therapy, 14,* 493–505.

Moore, M. L., Parsons, L., & Zaccaro, D. (1997). *Education, attitudes and practices of nurses from three practice sites concerning domestic violence.* Paper presented at the Eighth International Congress on Women's Health Issues, Saskatoon, Saskatchewan.

Morath, J. M., Casey, M., & Covert, E. (1985, Winter). The angry nurse/the angry staff. *Nursing Administration Quarterly,* pp. 45–49.

Morris, T., Greer, S., Pettingale, K., & Watson, M. (1981). Patterns of expression of anger and their psychological correlates in women with breast cancer. *Journal of Psychosomatic Research, 25,* 111–117.

Mozingo, J., Thomas, S., & Brooks, E. (1995). Factors associated with perceived competency levels of graduating seniors in a baccalaureate nursing program. *Journal of Nursing Education, 34,* 115–122.

Mrkwicka, L. (1994). Sexual harassment is no laughing matter. *International Nursing Review, 41*(4), 123–126.

Muff, J. (1988). *Women's issues in nursing: Socialization, sexism and stereotyping.* Prospect Heights, IL: Waveland Press. (Original work published 1982)

———. (1995). Hard refusals. *Perspectives in Psychiatric Care, 31*(3), 33–35.

Murray, R., & Zentner, J. P. (1979). *Nursing concepts for health promotion* (2nd ed.). Englewood Cliffs, NJ: Prentice-Hall.

Mynatt, S. (1996). A model of contributing risk factors to chemical dependency in nurses. *Journal of Psychosocial Nursing and Mental Health Services, 34*(7), 13–22.

Naisbett, J., & Aburdene, P. (1990). *Megatrends 2000.* New York: Morrow.

Nash, R. (1931). *A short life of Florence Nightingale.* New York: Macmillan.

Newsline. (1997). *American Psychological Association Monitor, 28*(8), 8.

Nightingale, F. (1992). *Notes on nursing: What it is and what it is not.* Philadelphia: Lippincott. (Original work published 1859)

Nolen-Hoeksema, S. (1987). Sex differences in unipolar depression: Evidence and theory. *Psychological Bulletin, 101,* 259–282.

———. (1990). *Sex differences in depression.* Stanford, CA: Stanford University Press.

Novaco, R. W. (1975). *Anger control: The development and evaluation of an experimental treatment.* Lexington, MA: Heath.

———. (1985). Anger and its therapeutic regulation. In M. A. Chesney & R. H. Rosenman (Eds.), *Anger and hostility in cardiovascular and behavioral disorders* (pp. 203–226). Washington, DC: Hemisphere.

———. (1996). Anger treatment and its special challenges. *National Center for PTSD Clinical Quarterly, 6*(3), 56, 58–60.

Nursing leadership in the 21st century: A report of ARISTA II. (1996). Indianapolis: Center Nursing Press, Sigma Theta Tau International.

Nursing shortage poll report. (1988, February). *Nursing,* pp. 33–41.

Ogus, E. D. (1990). Burnout and social support systems among ward nurses. *Issues in Mental Health Nursing, 11,* 267–281.

O'Leary, V. E., & Ickovics, J. R. (1994, May). *Women's resilience: A heuristic model.* Paper presented at the American Psychological Association Conference on Psychosocial and Behavioral Factors in Women's Health, Washington, DC.

O'Quinn-Larson, J. L. B. (1989). *Registered nurses' perceptions of factors related to chemical dependency in nursing students.* Unpublished doctoral dissertation, University of Texas, Austin.

Orbach, S. (1978). *Fat is a feminist issue.* New York: Paddington Press.

Orford, J., & Keddie, A. (1985). Gender differences in the functions and effects of moderate and excessive drinking. *British Journal of Clinical Psychology, 24,* 265–279.

Ornish, D. (1990). *Dr. Dean Ornish's program for reversing heart disease.* New York: Ballantine.

Peden, A. R. (1996). Recovering from depression: A one-year follow-up. *Journal of Psychiatric and Mental Health Nursing, 3,* 289–295.

Pelz, D. C., & Andrews, F. M. (1966). *Scientists in organization: Productive climates for research and development.* New York: Wiley.

Pennebaker, J. W. (1992). Inhibition as the linchpin of health. In H. S. Friedman (Ed.), *Hostility, coping, and health* (pp. 127–139). Washington, DC: American Psychological Association.

Perini, C., Muller, F., & Buhler, F. (1991). Suppressed aggression accelerates early development of essential hypertension. *Journal of Hypertension, 9,* 499–503.

Perls, F., Hefferline, R., & Goodman, P. (1951). *Gestalt therapy.* New York: Dell.

Peters, T. (1987). *Thriving on chaos.* Los Angeles: Excel.

Pew Health Professions Commission. (1993). *Health professions education for the future: Schools in service to the nation.* San Francisco: Author.

Pieranunzi, V. R. (1997). The lived experience of power and powerlessness in psychiatric nursing: A Heideggerian hermeneutical analysis. *Archives of Psychiatric Nursing, 11,* 155–162.

Plas, J. M., & Hoover-Dempsey, K. V. (1988). *Working up a storm.* New York: Norton.

Podrasky, D., & Sexton, D. (1988). Nurses' reactions to difficult patients. *Image, 20,* 16–21.

Polster, M. (1992). *Eve's daughter: The forbidden heroism of women.* San Francisco: Jossey-Bass.

Powell, L., Shaker, L., Jones, B., Vaccarino, L., Thoreson, C., & Pattillo, J. (1993). Psychosocial predictors of mortality in 83 women with premature acute myocardial infarction. *Psychosomatic Medicine, 55,* 426–433.

Powell, L., & Thoreson, C. (1987). Modifying the Type A pattern: A small group treatment approach. In J. A. Blumenthal & D. C. McKee (Eds.), *Applications in behavioral medicine and health psychology: A clinician's source book* (pp. 171–207). Sarasota, FL: Professional Resource Exchange.

Pratt, J. P., Overfield, T., & Hilton, H. G. (1994). Health behaviors of nurses and general population women. *Health Values, 18*(5), 41–46.

Progoff, I. (1975). *At a journal workshop: The basic text and guide for using the intensive journal process.* Dialogue House Library.

Radloff, L. (1975). Sex differences in depression: The effects of occupation and marital status. *Sex Roles, 1,* 249–265.

Ray, O., & Ksir, C. (1987). *Drugs, society, and human behavior.* St. Louis: Mosby.

Rein, G., Atkinson, M., & McCraty, R. (1995). The physiological and psychological effects of compassion and anger. *Journal of Advancement in Medicine, 8*(2), 87–105.

Remen, R. N. (1996). All emotions are potentially life affirming. *Advances: The Journal of Mind-Body Health, 12*(2), 25.

Reverby, S. (1987). *Ordered to care: The dilemma of American nursing, 1850–1945.* Cambridge: Cambridge University Press.

Rew, L., & Christian, B. (1993). Self-efficacy, coping, and well-being among nursing students sexually abused in childhood. *Journal of Pediatric Nursing, 8,* 392–399.

Reynolds, D. (1987). *Water bears no scars.* New York: Morrow.

Riley, W., Treiber, F., & Woods, M. (1989). Anger and hostility in depression. *Journal of Nervous and Mental Disease, 177,* 668–674.

Roberts, J. D. (1986). Games nurses play: Part 2. "Pass to a Higher Authority" and "Trivial Pursuit." *American Journal of Nursing, 86,* 945–956.

Roberts, S. (1991). Nurse abuse: A taboo topic. *Canadian Nurse, 87*(3), 23–25.

Roberts, S. J. (1983). Oppressed group behavior: Implications for nursing. *Advances in Nursing Science, 5*(7), 21–30.

Robbins, I., Bender, M. P., & Finnis, S. J. (1997). Sexual harassment in nursing. *Journal of Advanced Nursing, 25*(1), 163–169.

Rodgers, J. A. (1982). Women and the fear of being envied. *Nursing Outlook, 30,* 344–347.

Rosenblatt, R. (1997). Speech for a high school graduate. *Time, 149*(23), 90.

Rosenman, R. H., Brand, R. J., Jenkins, C. D., Friedman, M., Strauss, R., & Wurm, M. (1975). Coronary heart disease in the Western Collaborative Group Study: Final follow-up experience of 8½ years. *Journal of the American Medical Association, 233,* 872–877.

Ross, C. E., & Mirowsky, J. (1988). Child care and emotional adjustment to wives' employment. *Journal of Health and Social Behavior, 29,* 127–138.

Rothenberg, A. (1973). The anatomy of anger. In D. Carr & E. S. Casey (Eds.), *Explorations in phenomenology* (pp. 351–366). The Hague, Netherlands: Martinus Nijhoff.

Rubin, L. (1996). *The transcendent child: Tales of triumph over the past.* New York: Basic Books.

Ruiz, M. J. (1988). Lack of ego differentiation. In J. Muff (Ed.), *Women's issues in nursing: Socialization, sexism and stereotyping* (pp. 307–314). Prospect Heights, IL: Waveland Press.

Russell, S., & Shirk, B. (1993). Women's anger and eating. In S. P. Thomas (Ed.), *Women and anger* (pp. 170–185). New York: Springer.

Rutter, P. (1996). *Sex, power, and boundaries.* New York: Bantam.

Safran, J., & Greenberg, L. (1991). *Emotion, psychotherapy, and change.* New York: Guilford.

SAMHSA. (1995). *Substance abuse and mental health statistics sourcebook.* DHHS Publication No. (SMA) 95-3064. Washington, DC: U.S. Government Printing Office.

Sandelowski, M. (1986). The problem of rigor in qualitative research. *Advances in Nursing Science, 8,* 27–37.

Sandroff, R. (1982). Hooked: The story of one RN's battle with drugs. *RN, 46*(6), 45–47.

Sanford, J. A. (1977). *Healing and wholeness.* New York: Paulist Press.

Sanford, L. T., & Donovan, M. E. (1985). *Women and self-esteem.* New York: Penguin.

Sardana, R. M. (1997). *Bereavement in aging women: Psychosocial and cultural issues.* Paper presented at the Eighth International Congress on Women's Health Issues, Saskatoon, Saskatchewan.

Saussy, C. (1995). *The gift of anger: A call to faithful action.* Louisville, KY: Westminster John Knox Press.

Saylor, M., & Denham, G. (1993). Women's anger and self-esteem. In S. P. Thomas (Ed.), *Women and anger* (pp. 91–111). New York: Springer.

Schaub, B., & Schaub, R. (1997). *Healing addictions: The vulnerability model of recovery.* Albany, NY: Delmar.

Scherwitz, L., & Rugulies, R. (1992). Life-style and hostility. In H. S. Friedman (Ed.), *Hostility, coping and health* (pp. 77–98). Washington, DC: American Psychological Association.

Schilder, E. (1997, June). *The impact of organizational downsizing and restructuring on the worklife of nurses on acute medical wards in a tertiary care hospital.* Paper presented at the Eighth Congress of the International Council on Women's Health Issues, Saskatoon, Saskatchewan.

Schildmeier, D. (1997). Using public opinion to protect nursing practice. *American Journal of Nursing, 97*(3), 56–58.

Schrader, G. (1973). Anger and inter-personal communication. In D. Carr & E. Casey (Eds.), *Explorations in phenomenology* (pp. 331–350). The Hague, Netherlands: Martinus Nijhoff.

Schraeder, C., Lamb, G., Shelton, P., & Britt, T. (1997). Community nursing organizations: A new frontier. *American Journal of Nursing, 97*(1), 63–65.

Schuckit, M. A. (1989). *Drug and alcohol abuse: A clinical guide to diagnosis and treatment* (3rd ed.). New York: Plenum.

Schwartz, G., Weinberger, D., & Singer, J. (1981). Cardiovascular differentiation of happiness, sadness, anger, and fear following imagery and exercise. *Psychosomatic Medicine, 43,* 343–364.

Schwartz, J., Warren, K., & Pickering, T. (1994). Mood, location, and physical position as predictors of ambulatory blood pressure and heart rate: Application of a multi-level random effects model. *Annals of Behavioral Medicine, 16,* 210–220.

Seabrook, L. (1993). Women's anger and substance use. In S. P. Thomas (Ed.), *Women and anger* (pp. 186–208). New York: Springer.

Secunda, V. (1994, July). Victim trap. *New Woman,* 91–95.

Seldes, G. (1985). *The great thoughts.* New York: Ballantine.

Seligman, M. E. P. (1991). *Learned optimism.* New York: Knopf.

Seppa, N. (1996). "Charlie's Angels" made a negative, lasting impression. *American Psychological Association Monitor, 26*(4), 9.

―――. (1997). Children's TV remains steeped in violence. *American Psychological Association Monitor, 28*(6), 36.

Shapiro, D. H. (1982). Overview: Clinical and physiological comparison of meditation with other self-control strategies. *American Journal of Psychiatry, 139,* 267–273.

Shapiro, D., Schwartz, C., & Astin, J. (1996). Controlling ourselves, controlling our world: Psychology's role in understanding positive and negative consequences of seeking and gaining control. *American Psychologist, 51,* 1213–1230.

Shimer, C. (1997). Unlicensed and unsafe. *American Journal of Nursing, 97*(2), 19.

Shindul-Rothschild, J., Berry, D., & Long-Middleton, E. (1996). Where have all the nurses gone? Final results of our patient care survey. *American Journal of Nursing, 96*(11), 25–39.

Shoffner, D. (1997). Unlicensed assistive personnel: Helpful or harmful. *Tennessee Nurse, 60*(2), 13–15.

Siegman, A. W. (1994). From Type A to hostility to anger: Reflections on the history of coronary-prone behavior. In A. W. Siegman & T. W. Smith (Eds.), *Anger, hostility, and the heart* (pp. 1–21). Hillsdale, NJ: Erlbaum.

Siegman, A. W., Anderson, R. W., & Berger, T. (1990). The angry voice: Its effects on the experience of anger and cardiovascular reactivity. *Psychosomatic Medicine, 52,* 631–643.

Siegman, A. W., & Boyle, S. (1992). *The expression of anger and cardiovascular reactivity in men and women: An experimental investigation.* Paper presented at the meeting of the American Psychosomatic Society, New York.

Siegman, A. W., Dembroski, T. M., & Ringel, N. (1987). Components of hostility and the severity of coronary artery disease. *Psychosomatic Medicine, 49,* 127–135.

Simms, L. M., Erbin-Roesemann, M., Darga, A., & Coeling, H. (1990). Breaking the burnout barrier: Resurrecting work excitement in nursing. *Nursing Economics, 8*(3), 177–187.

Slaby, R., & Guerra, N. (1988). Cognitive mediators of aggression in adolescent offenders. *Developmental Psychology, 24,* 580–588.

Smith, F. (1981). Florence Nightingale: Early feminist. *American Journal of Nursing, 81,* 1021–1024.

―――. (1982). *Florence Nightingale: Reputation and power.* London: Croom Helm.

Smith, M., Droppleman, P., & Thomas, S. P. (1996). Under assault: The experience of work-related anger in female registered nurses. *Nursing Forum, 31*(1), 22–33.

Smith, M. E., & Hart, G. (1994). Nurses' responses to patient anger: From disconnecting to connecting. *Journal of Advanced Nursing, 20,* 643–651.

Solomon, R. (1976). *The passions.* Garden City, NY: Anchor Doubleday.

Sosne, D. (1996). Dangerous experiment with human subjects. *American Journal of Nursing, 96*(11), 41–42.

Spencer, J. (1982). *Becoming a nurse and a cigarette smoker: The first two years.* Institute of Nursing Studies, University of Hull.

Spiegel, D., Bloom, J. R., Kraemer, H. C., & Gottheil, E. (1989, October). Effect of psychosocial treatment on survival of patients with metastatic breast cancer. *The Lancet,* 888–891.

Spielberger, C. D. (1988). *State-Trait Anger Expression Inventory.* Orlando, FL: Psychological Assessment Resources.

Staff nurse guide to work redesign. (1997). *Tennessee Nurse, 60*(2), 16, 25.

Stapley, J., & Haviland, J. (1989). Beyond depression: Gender differences in normal adolescents' emotional experiences. *Sex Roles, 20,* 295–308.

Stein, L. (1967). The doctor-nurse game. *Archives of General Psychiatry, 16,* 699–703.

Stein, L., Watts, D., & Howell, T. (1990). The doctor-nurse game revisited. *New England Journal of Medicine, 322,* 546–549.

Steinem, G. (1991). *Revolution from within: A book of self-esteem.* Boston: Little, Brown.

Steingarten, J. (1994, August). Fancy that. *Vogue,* pp. 265, 303.

Stevick, E. L. (1971). An empirical investigation of the experience of anger. In A. Giorgi, W. F. Fischer, & R. Von Eckartsberg (Eds.), *Phenomenological psychology* (Vol. 1, pp. 132–148). Pittsburgh, PA: Duquesne University Press.

Stokols, D. (1992). Conflict-prone and conflict-resistant organizations. In H. S. Friedman (Ed.), *Hostility, coping and health* (pp. 65–76). Washington, DC: American Psychological Association.

Stoto, M. A. (1986). *Changes in adult smoking behavior in the United States: 1955–1983.* (Discussion Paper Series). Cambridge, MA: Institute for the Study of Smoking Behavior and Policy.

Strachey, L. (1996). *Florence Nightingale.* London: Penguin Books. (Original work published 1918)

Stratman, C. (1990). The experience of personal power for women. *Dissertation Abstracts International, 50,* 5896B.

Straus, M. A., & Gelles, R. (1987). The costs of family violence. *Public Health Reports, 102,* 638–641.

Suarez, E. C., & Williams, R. B. (1989). Situational determinants of cardiovascular and emotional reactivity in high and low hostile men. *Psychosomatic Medicine, 51,* 404–418.

————. (1990). The relationship between dimensions of hostility and cardiovascular reactivity as a function of task characteristics. *Psychosomatic Medicine, 52,* 558–570.

Suarez, E. C., Williams, R. B., Kuhn, C. M., & Schanberg, S. M. (1990, March). *Hostility scores predict cardiovascular, neurohormonal, and testosterone responses to harassment.* Paper presented at the meeting of the Society of Behavioral Medicine, Chicago.

Substance Abuse and Mental Health Services Administration, Office of Applied Studies (1994). *Preliminary estimates from the 1993 National Household Survey on Drug Abuse (NHSDA)* (Advance Report No. 7). Washington, DC: U.S. Government Printing Office.

Sullivan, J., & Deane, D. (1994). Caring: Reappropriating our tradition. *Nursing Forum, 29*(2), 5–9.

Survey finds consumer confidence in health care system eroding. (1997). *Capital Update, 15*(1), 5.

Tafrate, R. C. (1995). Evaluation of treatment strategies for adult anger disorders. In H. Kassinove (Ed.), *Anger disorders: Definition, diagnosis, and treatment* (pp. 109–129). Washington, DC: Taylor & Francis.

Tannen, D. (1994). *Talking from 9 to 5.* New York: Morrow.

Tavris, C. (1982). *Anger: The misunderstood emotion.* New York: Simon & Schuster.

————. (1989). *Anger: The misunderstood emotion* (rev. ed.). New York: Simon & Schuster.

Temoshok, L. (1985). Biopsychosocial studies on cutaneous malignant melanoma: Psychosocial factors associated with prognostic indicators, progression, psychophysiology, and tumor-host response. *Social Science and Medicine, 20,* 833–840.

Temoshok, L., & Dreher, H. (1992). *The Type C connection: The mind-body links to cancer and your health.* New York: Plume.

————. (1993, Spring). The Type C connection. *Noetic Sciences Review,* pp. 21–26.

Theorell, T., & Lind, E. (1973). Systolic blood pressure, serum cholesterol, and smoking in relation to sociological factors and myocardial infarction. *Journal of Psychosomatic Research, 17,* 327–332.

The war against women. (1994, March 28). *U.S. News and World Report,* p. 44.

Thomas, C. B. (1988). Cancer and the youthful mind: A forty-year perspective. *Advances: Journal of the Institute for the Advancement of Health, 5*(2), 42–58.

Thomas, L. (1996, December 3). "Re-engineering" is new term for describing when workers get the shaft. *Knoxville News-Sentinel,* p. C6.

Thomas, S. P. (1980). The adventures of Joey in patientland: A futuristic fantasy. *Nursing Forum, 19*(4), 350–356.

————. (1982). How to conduct an assertion training course for nursing students: A step-by-step plan for instruction. *Journal of Nursing Education, 21*(3), 33–37.

————. (1989). Gender differences in anger expression: Health implications. *Research in Nursing and Health, 12,* 389–398.

————. (1993a). The view from Scutari: A look at contemporary nursing. *Nursing Forum, 28*(2), 19–24.

————. (Ed.). (1993b). *Women and anger.* New York: Springer.

————. (1995). Women's anger: Causes, manifestations, and correlates. In C. D. Spielberger & I. G. Sarason (Eds.), *Stress and emotion: Anxiety, anger, and curiosity* (Vol. 15, pp. 53–74). Washington, DC: Taylor & Francis.

————. (1996). Nurse psychologists: A unique group within health psychology. *Journal of Clinical Psychology in Medical Settings, 3*(2), 93–101.

————. (1997a). Angry? Let's talk about it! *Applied Nursing Research, 10*(2), 80–85.

————. (1997b). Women's anger: Relationship of suppression to blood pressure. *Nursing Research, 46,* 324–330.

Thomas, S. P., & Donnellan, M. M. (1993). Stress, role responsibilities, social support, and anger. In S. P. Thomas (Ed.), *Women and anger* (pp. 112–128). New York: Springer.

Thomas, S. P., & Droppleman, P. (1997). Channeling nurses' anger into positive interventions. *Nursing Forum, 32*(2), 13–21.

Thomas, S. P., & Jozwiak, J. (1990). Self-attitudes and behavioral characteristics of Type A and B female registered nurses. *Health Care for Women International, 11,* 477–489.

Thomas, S. P., Smucker, C., & Droppleman, P. (in press). It hurts most around the heart: A phenomenological exploration of women's anger. *Journal of Advanced Nursing.*

Thomas, S. P., & Williams, R. (1991). Perceived stress, trait anger, modes of anger expression, and health status of college men and women. *Nursing Research, 40,* 303–307.

Thorne, B. (1993). *Gender play: Girls and boys in school.* New Brunswick, NJ: Rutgers University Press.

Tice, D. (1990, June). *Self-regulation of mood: Some self-report data.* Paper presented at the Nags Head Conference on Self-Control of Thought and Emotion. Nags Head, NC.

Tice, D., & Baumeister, R. (1993). Controlling anger: Self-induced emotion change. In D. M. Wegner & J. W. Pennebaker (Eds.), *Handbook of mental control* (pp. 393–409). Englewood Cliffs, NJ: Prentice-Hall.

Tiller, W., McCraty, R., & Atkinson, M. (1996). Cardiac coherence: A new, noninvasive measure of autonomic nervous system order. *Alternative Therapies, 2*(1), 52–65.

Tirrell, C. D. (1994). Psychoactive substance disorders among health care professionals. *Plastic Surgical Nursing, 14*(3), 169–172.

Trafford, A. (1997, May 6). Seconding the motion. *Washington Post,* p. 6.

Tsai, S., & Crockett, M. S. (1993). Effects of relaxation training, combining imagery and meditation, on the stress level of Chinese nurses working in modern hospitals in Taiwan. *Issues in Mental Health Nursing, 14,* 51–66.

Turkington, C. (1985). What price friendship? The darker side of social networks. *American Psychological Association Monitor, 16,* 38, 41.

Turner, R. J., & Avison, W. R. (1989). Gender and depression: Assessing exposure and vulnerability to life events in a chronically strained population. *Journal of Nervous and Mental Disease, 177,* 443–455.

U.S. Department of Health and Human Services. (1990a). *The health benefits of smoking cessation: A report of the Surgeon General.* Washington, DC: U.S. Government Printing Office.

U.S. Department of Health and Human Services. (1990b). *Health personnel in the United States: Seventh report to Congress.* Washington, DC: U.S. Government Printing Office.

Valentine, P. (1992). Feminism: A four-letter word? *The Canadian Nurse, 85*(12), 20–23.

Vasquez, J. (1997). Michigan program helps acute-care nurses transition to other settings. *The American Nurse, 29*(3), 24.

Vessey, J., & Gennaro, S. (1992). Caging the pushmi-pullu. *Nursing Research, 41,* 67.

Viorst, J. (1986). *Necessary losses.* New York: Simon & Schuster.

Wahler, R. G., Cartor, P. G., Fleischman, J., & Lambert, W. (1993). The impact of synthesis teaching and parent training with mothers of conduct-disordered children. *Journal of Abnormal Child Psychology, 21,* 425–440.

Walen, S. R., DiGiuseppe, R., & Wessler, R. L. (1980). *A practitioner's guide to rational-emotive therapy.* New York: Oxford University Press.

Ward, D., & Mullender, A. (1991). Empowerment and oppression: An indissoluble pairing for contemporary social work. *Critical Social Policy, 11*(2), 21–30.

Watson, J. (1985). *Nursing: Human science and health care.* Norwalk, CT: Appleton-Century-Crofts.

———. (1988). *Nursing: Human science and human care.* New York: National League for Nursing.

Watson, M., Pettingale, K., & Greer, S. (1984). Emotional control and autonomic arousal in breast cancer patients. *Journal of Psychosomatic Research, 28,* 467–474.

Weidner, G., Istvan, J., & McKnight, J. D. (1989). Clusters of behavioral coronary risk factors in employed women and men. *Journal of Applied Social Psychology, 19,* 468–480.

Weiner, B. (1991). Metaphors in motivation and attribution. *American Psychologist, 46,* 921–930.

Weinstein, N. D. (1984). Why it won't happen to me: Perceptions of risk factors and susceptibility. *Health Psychology, 3,* 431–457.

Weissman, M., & Paykel, E. (1974). *The depressed woman.* Chicago: University of Chicago Press.

What really *makes nurses angry.* (1986, January). *RN,* 55–60.

Whybrow, P. (1997). Making sense of mania and depression. *Psychology Today, 30*(3), 34–36, 38, 71–72.

Williams, C. L. (1995). Hidden advantages for men in nursing. *Nursing Administration Quarterly, 19*(2), 63–70.

Williams, R. B., Haney, T. L., Lee, K. L., Kong, Y., Blumenthal, J. A., & Whalen, R. (1980). Type A behavior, hostility, and coronary atherosclerosis. *Psychosomatic Medicine, 42,* 539–549.

Williams, R. B., & Williams, V. (1993). *Anger kills.* New York: Times Books.

Williams, R. L., Pettibone, T. J., & Thomas, S. P. (1991). Naturalistic application of self-change practices. *Journal of Research in Personality, 25,* 167–176.

Wing, R., Koeske, R., Epstein, L., Norwalk, M., Gooding, W., & Becker, D. (1987). Long-term effects of modest weight loss in Type II diabetic patients. *Archives of Internal Medicine, 147,* 1749–1753.

Witkin, G. (1991). *The female stress syndrome.* New York: Newmarket Press.

Wolf, N. (1993). *Fire with fire.* Toronto: Random House of Canada.

Wolpe, J. (1958). *Psychotherapy by reciprocal inhibition.* Stanford, CA: Stanford University Press.

Woodham-Smith, C. (1951). *Florence Nightingale.* New York: McGraw-Hill.

Woodman, M. (1982). *Addiction to perfection: The still unravished bride.* Toronto: Inner City Books.

Worell, J. (1996). Opening doors to feminist research. *Psychology of Women Quarterly, 20,* 469–485.

Yapko, M. D. (1997). The art of avoiding depression. *Psychology Today, 30*(3), 37, 75.

York, C., & Fecteau, D. (1987). Innovative models for professional nursing practice. *Nursing Economics, 5*(4), 162–166.

Young, B. H. (1996). From the editor. *National Center for PTSD Clinical Quarterly, 6*(3), 57.

Zillman, D. (1988). Mood management: Using entertainment to full advantage. In L. Donohew, H. E. Sypher, & E. T. Higgins (Eds.), *Communication, social cognition, and affect* (pp. 147–171). Hillsdale, NJ: Erlbaum.

Index

⑤ *Springer Publishing Company*

Effective Approaches to Patient's Behavior, 5th Edition

A Guide for Health Care Professionals, Patients, and their Caregivers

Gladys B. Lipkin, ARNP, EdD, FAAN
Roberta G. Cohen, RN, MS, CS

"Lipkin and Cohen offer...a practical workable how-to...that is a constructive and easy to use guide...It's like having your favorite preceptor or mentor making excellent creative suggestions and providing supportive guidance just when you feel you've exhausted your own ideas."
—**Jacqueline Rose Hott,** *RN, CS, FAAN, PhD*
Dean and Professor emerita,, Adelphi University School of Nursing

This concise guide to understanding and managing mental health indicators is the reference of choice for non-mental health specialists in nursing and social work. This edition is expanded to include factors presented to professionals working in manaed care environments, including specific short-term, intermediate, and long-term care guidelines.

Partial Contents:

I: Overview • Health Professionals in a Changing Workplace • Interactions Between Nurses and Patients in Managed Care

II: Approaches to Specific Psychiatric Disorders • The Person with Suicidal Ideation • The Person with an Obsessive-Compulsive Disorder

III: Approaches to the Psychological Effects of Special Circumstances • The Person who is a Victim of Abuse • The Person with a Sexual or Reproductive Disorder

IV: Approaches to the Psychological Effects of Physical Illness • The Person with Coronary Heart Disease or Cerebrovascular Accident • The Person With a Terminally Illness

V: Working With Different Age Groups • Crisis Intervention in the Lifespan • The Aged Person

1998 382pp. (est.) 0-8261-7771-9 hardcover

536 Broadway, New York, NY 10012-3955 • (212) 431-4370 • Fax (212) 941-7842

⑤ *Springer Publishing Company*

Spirituality in Nursing
From Traditional to New Age
Barbara Stevens Barnum, RN, PhD, FAAN

In this thoughtful examination of the reemergence of spirituality as an important factor in nursing practice, the author traces nursing's involvement with spirituality from its historical ties with religion to the current interest in alternative health methods. New nursing theories that involve spirituality, such as those of Dossey, Newman, and Watson are described. And nursing trends are put in the larger context of trends in society and other disciplines, such as psychology, physics, and philosophy.

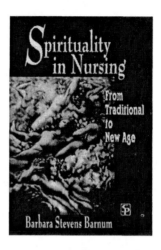

Contents:

- Spirituality in Nursing: Origins, Development, Overview
- Spirituality and Nursing's History
- Spirituality as a Component in Nursing Theory
- Developmental Theories: Is There a Spiritual Phase?
- Spirituality and the Emerging Paradigm
- Nursing Theorists in the New Paradigm
- Nursing and Healing
- Spirituality and Ethics: A Contrast in Forms
- Ethics and Philosophy
- Spirituality and the Mind
- Spirituality, Disease, and Death
- Spirituality and Religion
- Spiritual Therapeutics

1995   176pp   0-8261-9180-0   hardcover

536 Broadway, New York, NY 10012-3955 • (212) 431-4370 • Fax (212) 941-7842